ESSENTIAL CONCEPTS IN
IMMUNOLOGY

Irving L. Weissman
Stanford University

Leroy E. Hood
California Institute of Technology

William B. Wood
University of Colorado, Boulder

D1314967

The Benjamin/Cummings Publishing Company, Inc.
Menlo Park, California • Reading, Massachusetts
London • Amsterdam • Don Mills, Ontario • Sydney

Front cover photo: Lymphocytes and macrophages. [Courtesy of
J. Orenstein and E. Shelton.]

Other Books by the Authors

Biochemistry: A Problems Approach by Wood, Wilson, Benbow, and Hood
Molecular Biology of Eucaryotic Cells by Hood, Wilson, and Wood
Immunology by Hood, Weissman, and Wood

Sponsoring editor: Mary Forkner
Production editor: Margaret Moore
Editor: Jim Hall
Cover designer: Paul Quin
Artist: Georgeann Waggaman

Preface

Scope and Purposes of the Book

Essential Concepts in Immunology is a concise but comprehensive and up-to-date introduction to modern immunology. It has been designed for use as a textbook in introductory immunology courses or as a supplementary text in microbiology, pathology, or other courses that include immunology as part of their subject matter. The book is also intended as a convenient self-instruction text for health professionals who wish an up-to-date review of modern immunology and the biological bases of immune disease.

We have organized the subject matter of immunology into eight chapters.

Chapter 1 introduces the immune system and explains the dual nature of the protection it affords: cell-mediated immunity, provided by T-lymphocytes; and humoral immunity, provided by B-lymphocytes.

Chapter 2 begins with the biochemical and structural properties of antibodies, building from a simple exposition of their chemical structure to a more detailed discussion of antigen-recognizing and effector domains of immunoglobulin molecules of all classes. The latter part of this chapter considers the possible origins of antibody diversity and the organization of antibody genes in phylogeny and ontogeny.

Chapter 3 discusses the developmental biology of the immune system. It begins with the principles of clonal selection, and ends with a discussion of how lymphoid organs are organized in the most efficient manner to receive, recognize, and respond to antigenic stimulation.

Chapter 4 considers the immune response: the cellular, architectural, and molecular events that are triggered by antigenic stimulation. The function of each class and subclass of lymphoid cells and the antigen-induced interactions of these cells are discussed in detail. Also considered are the roles of cell-surface molecules coded by the major histocompatibility complex. The chapter closes with a description of how the immune response is regulated by feedback elements, by immune response genes, and by the self-nonself recognition mechanisms that are responsible for immunological tolerance.

Chapter 5 presents the most important immunochemical techniques and describes their application to modern immunoassay and immunodiagnosis.

Chapter 6 discusses the genetic, biochemical, and clinical principles of animal and human transplantation biology.

Chapter 7 considers the biological bases of immunological deficiency and immunological hypersensitivity diseases. It describes in detail the immunopathological consequences of abnormal immune responses to self and nonself antigens, and closes with the important new discoveries concerning the relationship of genes in the human major histocompatibility complex with clinically important immunological deficiency and hypersensitivity diseases.

Chapter 8 is devoted to cancer immunology. Beginning with a definition of cancer and the biological principles of tumor growth and carcinogenesis, this chapter then examines the hypothesis that cancer cells are antigenic and that the host responds to their antigenic determinants. The chapter closes with a discussion of the future prospects for immunotherapy and immunodiagnosis of cancer.

The material in each chapter is presented as a series of Essential Concepts, organized so as to present the most important general principles of each subject first, with more detailed information following in sub-paragraphs. To minimize difficulties with the complex terminology of immunology, each new term is clearly defined when first introduced, and jargon and abbreviations are avoided wherever possible. Numerous illustrations and photomicrographs are included to clarify the presentation. Following the Essential Concepts, each chapter includes a section of references and a series of true-false and fill-in exercises to help readers assess their understanding of the subject matter. Answers to these exercises appear at the end of the book. This organization of the text allows its use at several levels, from a quick scan of the Essential Concepts as a review of principles in modern immunology to a detailed study of the entire book for a more comprehensive introduction to the field.

Acknowledgments

Many people have helped with this book. We are indebted to Jonathan Howard and Allie Weissman for extensive criticism and helpful suggestions on Chapters 1–4, and to Barbara Birshtein, Henry Claman, Robert Fox, Jonathan Fuhrman, Carol Nottenburg, Bob Sanders, and Stewart Sell for reading and criticizing portions of the text. We are also indebted to Gerald Edelman, Sylvia Friedberg, George Gutman, Jan Orenstein, Robert Rouse, Willem van Ewijk, and Roger Warnke for making photomicrographs available. We thank the students and teaching assistants in our Caltech and Stanford immunology courses for their patience with early versions of the text and for their helpful suggestions. We are indebted to Jim Hall for creating the hospitable and productive environment of the Aspen Writing Center, and to Don King and the staff at the Given Institute of Pathology in Aspen for their generosity in allowing us to use their library facilities and participate in stimulating discussions with visitors at the Institute. Georgeann Waggaman skillfully transformed our crude drawings into finished artwork. Jim Hall, Mary Forkner, and Margaret Moore provided invaluable editorial help; Claire Wolf and members of the Caltech Biology Division typing pool contributed expert secretarial assistance. Finally, we appreciate the support and understanding of our families during the writing of this book.

I. Weissman, L. E. Hood, W. B. Wood

Contents

4 THE IMMUNE RESPONSE   41

5 IMMUNOASSAY AND IMMUNODIAGNOSIS   65

1 THE IMMUNE SYSTEM

Vertebrates possess a surveillance mechanism, called the immune system, that protects them from disease-causing (pathogenic) microorganisms, such as bacteria and viruses, and from cancer cells. The immune system specifically recognizes and selectively eliminates foreign invaders. Immunology, the study of the immune system, has contributed significantly to modern medicine in areas such as blood transfusion, vaccination, organ transplantation, and the treatment of allergy, autoimmune disease, and cancer. Immunology also has made vital contributions to cell biology by advancing our understanding of differentiation, cell-cell cooperation, and the triggering of proliferation and differentiation by cell-surface receptors. This chapter presents an overview of the immune system and its response to foreign invaders.

Essential Concepts

1-1 Two systems of immunity protect vertebrates

A. Immune protection in vertebrates is provided by a dual system that maintains two basic defenses against foreign invaders. Both systems respond specifically to most foreign substances, although one response generally is favored. The *cellular* immune response is particularly effective against fungi, parasites, intracellular viral infections, cancer cells, and foreign tissue. The *humoral* immune response defends primarily against the extracellular phases of bacterial and viral infections. Cellular immunity resides in cells of the lymphoid system. Humoral (circulating) immunity resides ultimately in the *serum*, which is the fluid phase of blood after cells and fibrinogen have been removed by clotting and centrifugation. Thus the two systems of immunity are distinct but provide overlapping protection.

B. The duality of the immune system results from two populations of morphologically indistinguishable lymphoid cells, called *lymphocytes*. Each lymphocyte in these two populations is poised to recognize and respond to one or a few closely related foreign substances.

1. One class of lymphocytes, the *T cells*, mediates the cellular immune response. When the organism is invaded by a foreign substance, T cells that recognize it are activated and initiate a reaction that eliminates the substance (Figure 1–1).

2. The other class of lymphocytes, the *B cells*, initiates the humoral immune response. Individual B cells, when activated by recognition of a foreign invader, differentiate to plasma cells which secrete *antibodies*, serum proteins that bind specifically to the foreign substance and initiate a variety of elimination responses (Figure 1–1).

C. In addition to lymphocytes, the immune system depends upon several other kinds of accessory cells (Figure 1–2). Their functions include trapping of foreign substances in the body for presentation to lymphocytes, scavenging of foreign invaders attacked by the immune system, and mediation of physiological changes that accompany the immune response.

D. The dual system of T- and B-cell immunity appears to be restricted to vertebrates. Specific cellular and humoral immune responses are found in bony fishes and even in the lowest vertebrates. The extent to which cellular and humoral immunity occur in invertebrates is still unclear, although efficient cellular scavenging mechanisms, transplant rejection, and potent inducible antibacterial substances have been demonstrated in several subvertebrate species.

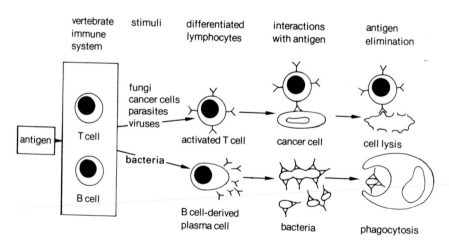

Figure 1–1 Differentiation, interaction, and elimination events that may occur upon stimulating T and B cells of the immune system.

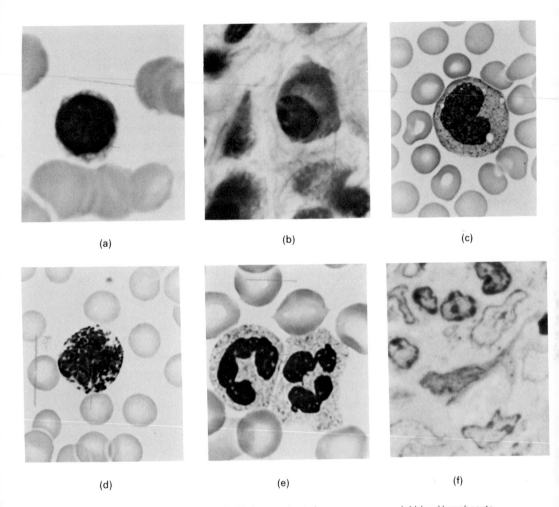

Figure 1-2 Cells associated with the vertebrate immune response: (a) blood lymphocyte (B or T), (b) plasma cell, (c) blood monocyte, (d) basophile, (e) polymorphonuclear leukocytes, (f) dendritic reticular cell. [Photomicrographs (a)–(e) courtesy of R. Rouse; (f) courtesy of G. Levine.]

1-2   The immune system recognizes foreign entities by their molecular features

A.   The essence of the immune system is its capacity to recognize surface features of macromolecules that are not normal constituents of the organism. The serum proteins called antibodies carry out this specific recognition, as do apparently similar molecules on the surfaces of T lymphocytes. The foreign entities that these agents recognize are termed *antigens*. The portion of an antigen to which an antibody binds is called an *antigenic determinant* (Figure 1–3). Antibodies recognize

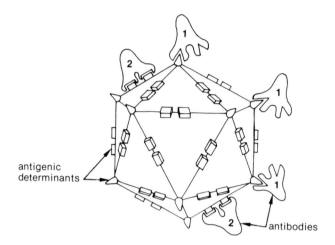

Figure 1–3 A virus interacting with antibodies specific for two types of antigenic determinants.

and bind antigens by molecular complementarity, which permits multiple noncovalent interactions of the same types that confer specificity on enzyme–substrate binding. An antigen complementary to a specific antibody is called a *cognate* antigen.

B. An antigen that elicits a response from the immune system is referred to as an *immunogen*. Macromolecules such as foreign proteins, nucleic acids, and carbohydrates usually are effective immunogens; molecules with molecular weights of less than 5000 usually are not. However, many small nonimmunogenic molecules, termed *haptens*, can stimulate an immune response if covalently attached to a large *carrier* molecule. For example, the 2,4-dinitrophenyl group rarely is immunogenic unless attached to a carrier protein such as serum albumin (Figure 1–4).

Animals that have an appropriate number of activated specific T cells or an appropriate concentration of specific antibody in their blood are *immune* to the cognate antigens.

C. Antibodies belong to a class of proteins called *immunoglobulins*. The basic unit of immunoglobulin structure is a complex of four polypeptides, two identical "light" (low molecular weight) chains and two identical "heavy" (high molecular weight) chains, linked together by disulfide bonds (Figure 1–5).

The carboxyl-terminal (C-terminal) portions of the light and heavy chains, termed the *constant* regions, are nearly identical for antibodies of the same class. The stem of an immunoglobulin molecule, formed by the C-terminal halves of the two heavy chains, is called the *Fc*

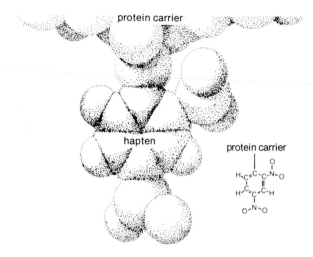

Figure 1–4 Three-dimensional representation of a simple hapten, the dinitrophenyl group, attached to a hypothetical protein carrier. The structural formula of the dinitrophenyl group is shown at the right. [Adapted from G. Edelman, *Sci. Am.* **223,** 34 (1970). Copyright © 1970 by Scientific American, Inc. All rights reserved.]

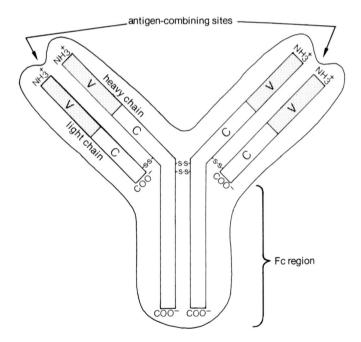

Figure 1–5 A two-dimensional representation of the antibody molecule. The heavy and light chains are joined by disulfide bridges. The N-terminal (NH_3^+) and C-terminal (COO^-) ends and the variable (V) and constant (C) regions of each chain are oriented as shown. The envelope around the molecule approximates its three-dimensional shape, with the antigen-combining sites indicated.

region. The amino-terminal (N-terminal) portions of the light and heavy chains differ substantially in amino-acid sequence between individual species of antibody. These *variable* regions of the light and heavy chains combine to form the antigen binding sites of an antibody molecule, as shown in Figure 1–5. The *valence* of an antibody is the number of identical antigen-binding sites per molecule. The *affinity* of an antibody-combining site is a measure of the strength of its binding to an antigenic determinant. The term *avidity* is used to describe the net strength of interaction of a *multivalent* antibody with a *multideterminant* antigen.

1. The variable and constant regions, respectively, are responsible for the two functions of an antibody: the *antigen-recognition function* and the *effector function.* Circulating antibodies have a variety of characteristic effector functions that are involved in the elimination of foreign antigens.

2. Immunoglobulins in mammalian serum can be divided into five classes on the basis of amino-acid-sequence differences in the constant regions of their heavy chains. These classes, designated IgM, IgG, IgA, IgD, and IgE, correspond to antibodies with different effector functions.

Selected Bibliography

Burnet, F. M. (Ed.), *Immunology,* W. H. Freeman and Company, San Francisco, 1976. A collection of articles reprinted from *Scientific American* on many different aspects of immunology.

Jerne, N. K., "The immune system," *Sci. Am.* **229,** 52 (1973).

Exercises

1–1 Indicate whether each of the following statements is true or false. Explain the error in each statement you consider to be false.

(a) An antibody molecule has one type of antigen-binding site.

(b) A large antigen generally can combine with many different antibody molecules.

(c) Immunogenic antigens stimulate production of antibodies that recognize them.

F (d)   A hapten can stimulate antibody production but cannot combine with antibody molecules.

T (e)   Both the cellular and humoral responses play a role in host defense against viral infections.

F (f)   T cells secrete antibody molecules.

F (g)   The C-terminal halves of the light chains constitute the Fc region of the antibody molecule.

T (h)   The valence of the antibody molecule depicted in Figure 1–5 is two.

1–2   Supply the missing word or words in each of the following statements.

(a)   When haptens are attached to a larger _Carrier_ molecule, they become immunogenic.

(b)   _Plasma cells_ are the terminal effector cells of B-cell differentiation.

(c)   T cells mediate _cellular_ immunity.

(d)   _Humoral_ immunity is protective against extracellular bacterial infections.

(e)   The effector functions of an immunoglobulin are defined by the class of its _heavy_ chains.

(f)   The presence of specific immunoglobulin responses to antigen in the animal kingdom is thought to be limited to _vertebr_.

(g)   An antigen complementary to a specific antibody is called a _cognate_ antigen.

(h)   The five major classes of immunoglobulins are _IgM_, _IgG_, _IgA_, _IgD_, and _IgE_.

Answers are given on page 154.

2 ANTIBODIES

The antibody molecule has evolved to perform two distinct functions—antigen recognition and elimination. Antibody molecules can interact with a virtually unlimited number of antigens, yet antibodies destroy or eliminate antigens by a small number of effector mechanisms. To carry out its dual function the antibody has evolved discrete molecular domains. One of these domains binds antigen, and the others mediate effector functions. Thus the functional duality of the antibody molecule is reflected in its three-dimensional structure. The organization of antibody gene families also reflects this functional duality. These gene families must be capable of storing or generating information for hundreds of thousands of different antibody molecules. This chapter considers the structure and function of antibody molecules.

Essential Concepts

2-1 Immunoglobulin structure is known from studies of myeloma proteins

A. The serum of a normal vertebrate contains a large variety of proteins, including the five classes of immunoglobulins (Figure 2–1). The immunoglobulins in turn include the organism's circulating antibody population. The basic structures and gross chemical properties of immunoglobulins are very similar, but their combining specificities vary widely, reflecting the spectrum of antigens that the individual has encountered during its lifetime.

The immunoglobulins are so similar and yet normally so heterogeneous that isolation of an individual molecular species for detailed chemical study is difficult. Fortunately, homogeneous immunoglobulins can be obtained by taking advantage of an abnormal condition, a cancer of antibody-producing cells called *multiple myeloma*. In an individual afflicted with this disease, neoplastic transformation generally occurs in a single plasma cell or its immediate precursor, so that the resulting

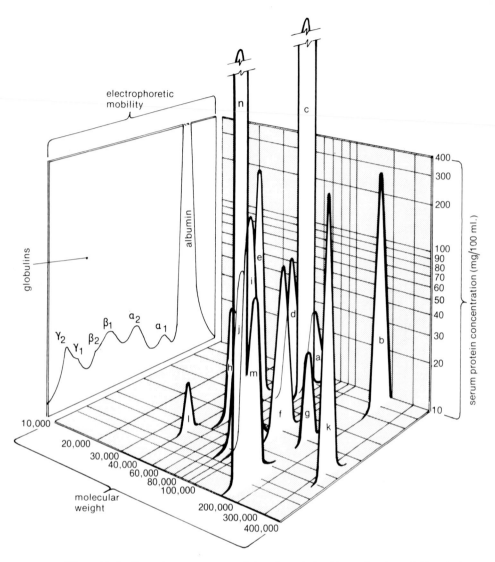

Figure 2-1 Some human serum proteins characterized by molecular weights, electrophoretic mobilities at pH 8.6, and concentrations in the blood serum. For purposes of comparison, the mobilities and concentrations of the globulins (α, β, γ) and albumin are shown at the rear. Proteins are identified by the following letters: a, prealbumin; b, α_1 lipoprotein; c, albumin; d, α_1 acid glycoprotein; e, α_1 antitrypsin; f, haptoglobulin; g, ceruloplasm; h, α_2 HS glycoprotein; i, transferrin; j, hemopexin; k, fibrinogen; l, β_2 glycoprotein; m, IgA; n, IgG.

tumor secretes a homogeneous immunoglobulin (*myeloma protein*). This protein can comprise 95% of the serum immunoglobulin, and therefore is easy to isolate in pure form. The myeloma protein from any afflicted individual generally is different from myeloma proteins in all other afflicted individuals. Myeloma tumors have been observed in many mammalian species, including man, rat, mouse, horse, and dog.

B.   Myeloma proteins are indistinguishable from normal immuno-globulins by all available criteria. All the types of polypeptide chains and genetic markers seen in normal immunoglobulins have been found in myeloma proteins. Extensive amino-acid sequences are identical in normal and myeloma immunoglobulins. Some myeloma proteins bind known antigenic determinants. These myeloma proteins have structures that are identical to their normal counterparts induced by immunization with the appropriate hapten. These observations suggest that myeloma proteins are similar, if not identical, to normal antibody molecules.

2-2   Immunoglobulin molecules are composed of two kinds of polypeptides

A.   Immunoglobulin molecules of the most common class, IgG, are made up of two identical light chains of molecular weight 23,000 and two identical heavy chains of molecular weight 53,000 (Figure 2–2). Each light chain is linked to a heavy chain by noncovalent associations and also by one covalent disulfide bridge. In the IgG molecule the two light chain–heavy chain (L–H) pairs are linked together by disulfide

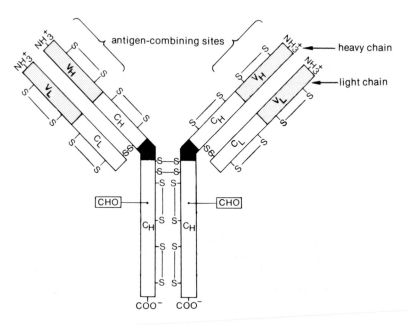

Figure 2–2 A schematic drawing of the human immunoglobulin G (IgG) molecule, showing its principal structural features. Dark portions of the two heavy chains indicate the hinge region. V regions are indicated by shaded segments. The remainder of each polypeptide is the C region. V and C indicate regions of variable and constant amino-acid sequence, respectively, as explained in Essential Concept 2–3. Loops are the result of 12 intrachain disulfide bridges at the positions shown. Two interchain disulfide bridges are in the hinge region. CHO represents carbohydrate groups attached to the heavy chains.

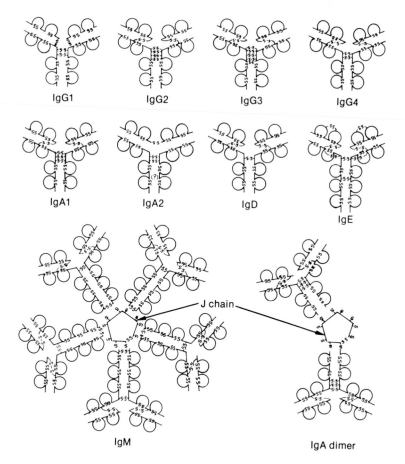

Figure 2–3 Subunit structures of various human immunoglobulins. —S—S— indicates a disulfide bridge. The question mark indicates that the interchain disulfide bridge structure is unknown. IgG1, IgG2, IgG3, and IgG4 are subclasses of IgG. IgA1 is the monomeric subclass of the IgA class. The J chain joins the subunits in the multimeric forms of IgA as well as the five subunits of the IgM molecule. [Adapted from J. Gally in *The Antigens*, M. Sela (Ed.), Academic Press, New York, 1973, p. 209.]

bridges between the heavy chains. As shown in Figure 2–2, the molecule can be represented schematically in the form of a Y, with the amino (N−) termini of the four chains at the top and the carboxyl (C−) termini of the two heavy chains at the bottom. The portion of the molecule that includes the disulfide linkages between heavy chains where the three arms of the Y come together is called the hinge region.

The arms of the Y are flexible. Twelve intrachain disulfide bridges are spaced periodically, two in each light chain and four in each heavy chain. Carbohydrate groups are attached through the side chains of asparagine residues in the two heavy chains at the positions shown in Figure 2–2. Thus immunoglobulins are glycoproteins.

B. A dimer of light chain–heavy chain pairs, $(L-H)_2$, is the basic structural subunit of other classes of immunoglobulin molecules as well as of IgG. The structures of other classes and subclasses differ in the positions and number of the disulfide bridges between heavy chains, and in the number of $(L-H)_2$ subunits in the molecule (Figure 2–3). IgD and IgE molecules, like IgG, are composed of one $(L-H)_2$ subunit. The IgA molecule may have one, two, or three $(L-H)_2$ subunits. The serum IgM molecule has five $(L-H)_2$ subunits, that is, it is equivalent to an aggregate of five IgG-like molecules. The membrane-bound IgM molecule has one $(L-H)_2$ subunit. In the higher polymeric forms of IgA and in IgM, the $(L-H)_2$ subunits are held together by disulfide bridges through a polypeptide called the *J chain.*

2–3   The polypeptides of immunoglobulins are differentiated into variable and constant regions

When the amino-acid sequences of several myeloma light chains first were compared, a striking pattern emerged (Figure 2–4). In the N-terminal half of the chain the sequences were found to vary greatly from polypeptide to polypeptide. By contrast, in the C-terminal half of the chain the sequences of all the molecules were identical. Consequently these two segments of the molecule were designated the *variable* (V_L) and *constant* (C_L) regions of the light chain, respectively. The V_L region begins at the N-terminus and is approximately 110 amino-acid residues in length. The C_L region makes up the remainder of the chain, and also is about 110 residues in length.

Heavy-chain sequences exhibit a similar pattern. A variable (V_H) region begins at the N-terminus and is approximately the same length

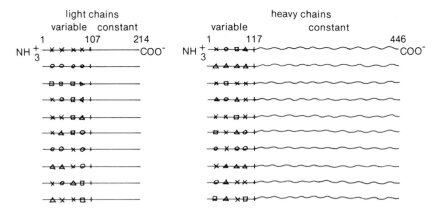

Figure 2–4 A schematic representation of the variable and constant regions for light and heavy chains from ten IgG molecules. NH_3^+ indicates the N-terminus and COO^- the C-terminus. x, O, △, and □ indicate amino-acid-sequence differences. Lines without these symbols indicate sequence identity among the proteins compared. The lengths of the V and C regions are indicated by residue number, beginning with Residue 1 at the N-terminus.

as the V_L region of the light chain, about 110 residues. The heavy-chain constant (C_H) region for the IgG molecule is about three times this length, or about 330 residues.

The V_L and V_H regions of each L–H pair comprise the antigen-binding sites in an immunoglobulin molecule (Figure 2–2). The C_H regions carry out effector functions, which are common to all antibodies of a given class. Each immunoglobulin molecule has at least two identical antigen-binding sites. This bivalence permits antibodies to cross-link antigens with two or more antigenic determinants. The flexibility of the arms of the antibody molecule allows it to bind simultaneously to antigenic determinants that are separated by various distances.

2-4   The antigen-binding site can exhibit a broad range of specificities

A.   The active site is a crevice between the V_L and V_H regions (Figure 2–5). The size and shape of the antigen-binding site can vary significantly from one antibody to another due to differences in the relationship of the V_L and V_H regions, and due to amino-acid-sequence variation in the V_L and V_H regions. Antibody specificity results from molecular complementarity between determinant groups on the antigen molecule and amino-acid residues in the active site.

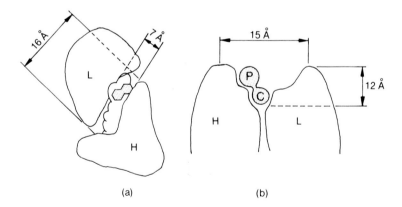

(a)   (b)

Figure 2–5   (a) A schematic top view of the shallow cleft between the heavy and light variable regions of the human myeloma protein NEW, which specifically binds the hapten, vitamin K_1OH (shaded). The dimensions of the binding site are 16 Å x 7 Å x 6 Å. [Redrawn from F. Richards *et al., The Immune System: Genes, Receptors, Signals,* E. Sercarz, A. Williamson, and C. Fox (Eds.), Academic Press, New York, 1975, p. 53.] (b) A schematic side view of the interaction of the variable regions of mouse myeloma protein McPC603 with its specific hapten, phosphorylcholine (shaded). The dimensions of the binding site are 20 Å x 15 Å x 12 Å. [Redrawn from E. Padlan *et al., The Immune System: Genes, Receptors, Signals,* E. Sercarz, A. Williamson, and C. Fox (Eds.), Academic Press, New York, 1975, p. 7.]

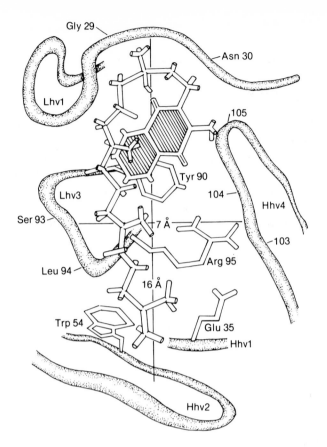

Figure 2–6 A schematic drawing of the hapten, vitamin K_1OH, bound to the combining site of a human IgG molecule. Lhv1, Lhv3, Hhv1, Hhv2, and Hhv4 designate the approximate locations of the hypervariable regions of the light and heavy chains, respectively. The quinone group (two fused six-membered rings) of the hapten is bound at the top in a shallow crevice (16Å x 7 Å x 6 Å); the phytyl tail folds over the quinone and extends along most of the length of the active site. [From I. M. Amzel *et al., Proc. Natl. Acad. Sci. USA* **71,** 1427 (1974).]

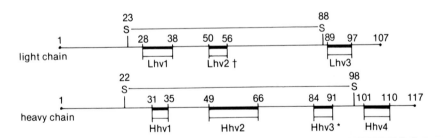

Figure 2–7 A linear map of hypervariable segments in the variable regions of light and heavy chains. Residue numbers indicate the approximate end points of these segments and the positions of central disulfide bridges. * indicates a hypervariable segment that is not part of the antigen-binding crevice (see Figure 2–6). † indicates a hypervariable segment that sometimes is a part of the antigen-binding crevice.

B.   The walls of the antigen-binding site are composed of *hypervariable* (hv) segments of the V_L and V_H regions (Figure 2–6). These regions of extensive diversity initially were defined by comparing immunoglobulin chains from a given class after alignment for sequence homology. Three hypervariable segments generally are present in V_L regions, and four in V_H regions (Figure 2–7).

C.   The antigen-binding sites of antibodies differ from the substrate-binding sites of most enzymes in one fundamental way: two chains, rather than one, fold to make the antigen-binding site. Thus extensive binding-site diversity can be generated by the combinatorial properties of light chain–heavy chain association in antibody synthesis (Figure 2–8). For example, if any light chain can associate with any heavy chain to produce a functional antibody, then 1000 different light chains and 1000 different heavy chains can be combined in pairs to produce $10^3 \times 10^3 = 10^6$ different antibody molecules. The combinatorial diversity increases as the product of the numbers of different available light and heavy chains.

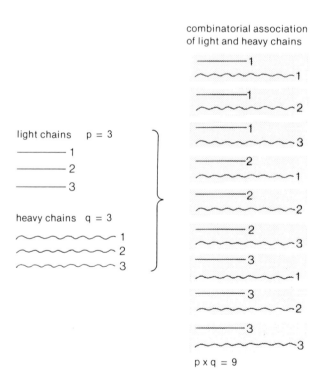

Figure 2–8   The generation of antigen-binding-site diversity by combinatorial association of three different light chains and three different heavy chains. The total number of different binding sites that can be generated from *p* light chains and *q* heavy chains is *p* × *q*.

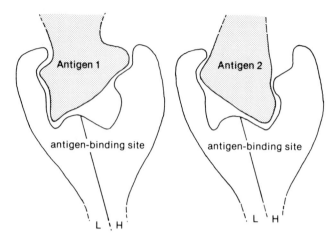

Figure 2–9   A schematic representation of multispecificity in a single antibody molecule.

D.   The diversity of antigen-binding capability is still further increased by a phenomenon called *multispecificity,* the ability of a single antibody molecule to combine with a spectrum of different antigens. Multispecificity is biologically significant. Because a particular antibody receptor can be triggered by different antigenic determinants, an organism can respond to completely novel antigens, including synthetic compounds never before encountered by the species.

Although a single antibody molecule has a unique three-dimensional structure, it can combine with the inducing antigenic determinant, determinants with similar structures (cross-reacting antigens), and perhaps even determinants with quite disparate structures. A stable antigen–antibody complex will result whenever there is a sufficient number of short-range interactions, regardless of the total fit. The antigen-combining site is large, and a lack of fit in one area can be compensated for by increased binding elsewhere. Therefore, disparate antigens may fit into the antigen-binding crevice in different ways (Figure 2–9). Each species of antibody has a different spectrum of determinants with which it can combine.

2–5   Homology units in immunoglobulins correspond to molecular domains with different functions

A.   On the basis of primary structure comparisons, light and heavy chains may be divided into two groups of *homology units* of similar amino-acid sequence (Figure 2–10). Each of these units is about 110 residues in length and has a centrally placed disulfide bridge. One group consists of the V_L and V_H regions. The other group consists of the

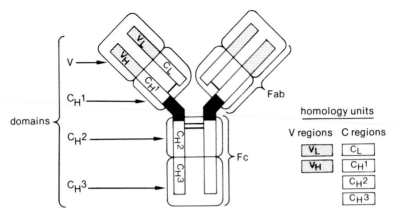

Figure 2–10 A diagrammatic representation of the homology units and domains of the IgG molecule. Pairs of homology units fold together to form four globular domains termed V, C_H1, C_H2, and C_H3, as indicated by boxes in the figure. Limited proteolytic attack at the hinge region (shaded segment of heavy chains) cleaves the molecule into Fab and Fc fragments.

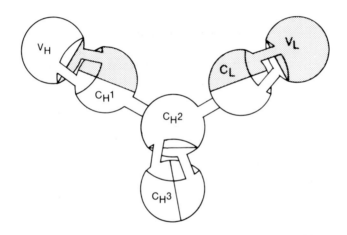

Figure 2–11 The domains of the human IgG molecule as determined by X-ray analysis at 6 Å. [Reproduced from R. J. Poljak *et al.*, *Nature* **235**, 137 (1972), Figure 3.]

C_L region and three subsegments of the C_H region, designated C_H1, C_H2, and C_H3.

The immunoglobulin molecule is folded into discrete, compact, globular domains connected by short segments of more extended polypeptide chain (Figure 2–11). Each domain consists of a pair of corresponding homology units folded together. The V_L and V_H homology units form the V domain; the C_L and C_H1 units form the C_H1 domain; two C_H2 units form the C_H2 domain; and two C_H3 units form the C_H3 domain (Figure 2–10). Thus the basic (L–H)$_2$ immunoglobulin unit is composed of six globular domains: two V, two C_H1, one C_H2, and one C_H3.

Proteolytic digestion under suboptimal conditions can cause limited cleavage of native immunoglobulin molecules between globular domains. Presumably the compactly folded domains are protected from proteolysis, whereas the regions of more extended polypeptide chain between homology units are accessible. Early experiments of this kind showed that the IgG molecule can be broken into two fragments by cleavage of the hinge region of the heavy chain (Figure 2–10). One fragment, which turned out to be readily crystallizable and consequently is designated the Fc fragment, consists of the C_H2 and C_H3 domains. The second fragment contains two identical subunits held together by a particularly labile disulfide bond; mild reduction yields two fragments. These two fragments, designated Fab (for *antigen-binding fragment*), are identical. Each consists of one V and one C_H1 domain, so that each carries one antigen-binding site.

B.   The antigen-binding functions and effector functions of immunoglobulins are carried out by different domains of the molecule. The V domains are responsible for antigen binding, whereas the C domains carry out the various effector functions.

2-6   The five classes of immunoglobulin molecules differ in the structures of their heavy-chain constant regions

A.   The five immunoglobulin classes are distinguished structurally by differences in their heavy-chain constant regions. Comparisons of C_H-region amino-acid sequences show that there are five major heavy-chain classes, designated α, γ, δ, ε, and μ. These heavy-chain classes define the corresponding immunoglobulin classes IgA, IgG, IgD, IgE, and IgM, respectively. Some classes can be divided into subclasses, defined by C_H regions that are distinct but more similar in amino-acid sequence; for example, the γ class can be divided into $\gamma1$, $\gamma2$, $\gamma3$, and $\gamma4$ subclasses. The genes that code for heavy chains are known collectively as the *heavy-chain (H) gene family.*

B.   In addition there are two major *types* of light chains based on C_L-region amino-acid-sequence comparisons. These two types are designated kappa (κ) and lambda (λ). Like some heavy-chain classes, the λ light-chain types may be further divided into subtypes defined by distinct but very similar C_L sequences. The genes that code for these light-chain types comprise the λ *gene family* and the κ *gene family,* respectively.

C.   The five classes of immunoglobulins are defined by the classes of their constituent heavy-chain subunits only (Table 2–1). The class of an immunoglobulin molecule is independent of the type of light-chain

Table 2–1
Subunit structures of the five immunoglobulin classes in humans

Class	Heavy chain	Subclasses	Light chain	Molecular formula
IgG	γ	$\gamma1, \gamma2$ $\gamma3, \gamma4$	κ or λ	$(\gamma_2\kappa_2)$ $(\gamma_2\lambda_2)$
IgA	α	$\alpha1, \alpha2$	κ or λ	$(\alpha_2\kappa_2)_n^a$ $(\alpha_2\lambda_2)_n$
IgM	μ	none	κ or λ	$(\mu_2\kappa_2)_5$ $(\mu_2\lambda_2)_5$
IgD	δ	none	κ or λ	$(\delta_2\kappa_2)$ $(\delta_2\lambda_2)$
IgE	ϵ	none	κ or λ	$(\epsilon_2\kappa_2)$ $(\epsilon_2\lambda_2)$

[a]n may equal 1, 2, or 3.

subunits that it contains. A single immunoglobulin molecule always has identical light and identical heavy chains; however, immunoglobulin molecules of a given class may contain either λ or κ light chains. The subunit compositions of the five immunoglobulin classes are listed in Table 2–1. Fully mature plasma cells invariably produce only a single species of heavy chain and a single species of light chain.

D.   Although all immunoglobulin molecules probably bind antigens in a similar fashion, the different classes serve different physiological functions. The functional differences of the five classes reflect the structural differences in their heavy-chain constant regions, which comprise the effector domains of all immunoglobulin molecules.

2-7   Two genes code for each immunoglobulin polypeptide chain

Recent studies employing the techniques of nucleic acid chemistry have established that the V and C regions are coded by separate genes. Since V and C regions are coded by separate genes, their information must be combined at either the DNA, the RNA, or the protein level to produce a complete immunoglobulin polypeptide. This V-C joining event appears to be a fundamental component in the differentiation of each antibody-producing cell. Thus the study of antibody genes may provide important general insights into the differentiation of other complex systems in eukaryotes.

2-8   The origin of antibody diversity is still debated

A.   The vertebrate immune system is capable of synthesizing perhaps 10^5 to 10^8 different antibody molecules, which collectively can recognize a virtually unlimited number of different antigens. How does an organism generate this vast antibody diversity? Many immunologists in the 1930's and 1940's favored the hypothesis that antigens could *instruct* the organism to make complementary antibodies by serving as templates around which antibody polypeptides might fold. However, the instructionist theories were ruled out in the early 1960's when it was shown that the folding of an antibody molecule can be determined entirely by its amino-acid sequence in the absence of antigen. Following this demonstration, attempts to explain antibody diversity became focused on the origin of amino-acid-sequence diversity in the V_L and the V_H regions.

B.   Two general theories have been put forward to explain the observed amino-acid-sequence diversity of light-chain and heavy-chain variable regions.

1.   The *germ-line theory* postulates that most, if not all V-region genes are separately encoded in the zygote or germ line of the organism. These genes are assumed to have arisen by gene duplication, mutation, and selection during vertebrate evolution. According to this theory, the diversity of V-region genes exists prior to the differentiation of each individual, and antibody synthesis requires merely the activation of preexisting antibody genes in each lymphocyte.

2.   The *somatic variation* theory postulates that V-region diversity develops from a relatively small number of germ-line genes, which diversify by some mutational process during development of the immune system. According to this theory, V-region diversity is generated anew in each individual rather than passed from one generation to the next.

Recent experimental data from studies of immunoglobulin amino-acid sequences and the nucleotide sequences that code for them suggest that both of these mechanisms may be employed by vertebrate immunity. These studies represent one of the most active areas of research in contemporary immunology.

Selected Bibliography

Edelman, G. M., "The structure and function of antibodies," *Sci. Am.* **223**, 34 (1970).

Kabat, E. A., *Structural Concepts in Immunology and Immunochemistry,* Holt, Rinehart, and Winston, New York, 1976. An up-to-date text with a comprehensive coverage of antibody structure.

Exercises

2–1   Indicate whether each of the following statements is true or false. Explain the error in each statement you consider to be false.

F   (a)   The hinge region joins light and heavy chains in the immunoglobulin molecule.

F   (b)   One immunoglobulin molecule can have light chains with two different V-region sequences.

F   (c)   The V_H region is twice the length of the V_L region.

T   (d)   Homology units of immunoglobulin polypeptides are encoded by nucleotide sequences of about 330 nucleotide pairs in length.

F   (e)   The immunoglobulin active site is composed primarily of the light chain.

F   (f)   IgG1 and IgG2 molecules are distinguished by differences in their C_L sequences.

F   (g)   A single antigen generally evokes the synthesis of a single molecular species of antibody.

(h)   Myeloma proteins from different humans always are identical in sequence.

T   (i)   The germ-line theory suggests that there are many V genes in the germ line.

2–2   Supply the missing word or words in each of the following statements.

(a)   The diversity of antigen-binding sites presumably reflects in the amino-acid-sequence diversity of the subunit ___V___ regions.

(b)   The _Somatic_ theory contends that the information content of the genome can be expanded during somatic differentiation.

(c)   _Myeloma_ are homogeneous immunoglobulins derived from organisms with plasma-cell tumors.

(d)   The IgG antibody molecule folds into six discrete _domains_.

(e)   The _hypervariable_ regions fold to form the walls of the antigen-binding crevice.

(f)   The _effector_ functions of immunoglobulins from different classes are different, whereas the _recogn_ function may be the same.

(g)   The two types of light chains are _kappa_ and _lambda_.

Answers are given on pages 154–155.

3 DEVELOPMENT AND ARCHITECTURE OF THE IMMUNE SYSTEM

The immune response depends upon a population of cells that collectively is capable of antigen processing, antigen recognition, intercellular communication, antigen-driven differentiation, and expression of effector functions. These cells are contained largely within a system of lymphoid organs, and are organized into compartments that maximize appropriate cellular interactions. This chapter considers the central participants in the immune response, immunologically competent T and B lymphocytes, in terms of their specificities, their embryologic origins, and their locations within lymphoid organs.

Essential Concepts

3-1 Each lymphocyte is predetermined to express membrane receptors with a single specificity for antigen

A. The general mechanism by which a vertebrate mounts a specific immune response to any of a nearly infinite variety of antigens was explained in the 1950's by the clonal selection theory of antibody formation, a set of postulates put forward by Jerne, Burnet, Lederberg, and Talmage. Subsequent research has substantiated these postulates, which are stated in their modern form in Sections B through E and are diagramed in Figure 3–1.

B. The cell surfaces of lymphocytes carry membrane-bound antibodies or antibody-like molecules that function as antigen receptors. The receptors of B cells are known to be antibodies, which are present on the membrane in a quantity of about 10^5 molecules per cell. The receptors of T cells appear to have similar properties, but their molecular nature is still unknown. Binding of an antigen to a B-cell receptor initiates a humoral immune response; binding to a T-cell initiates a cellular immune response.

Each lymphocyte carries only one kind of specific receptor; therefore, it will respond to only a few closely related antigenic determinants. All cells bearing a particular receptor are thought to belong to the same clone; that is, they are the progeny of a single ancestral cell with that receptor. A mature mammal contains 10^8 to 10^{12} lymphocytes, which collectively possess the capacity to respond to an enormous variety of antigens. This lymphocyte population is thought to consist of 10^5 to 10^8 clones of cells with different receptor specificities. Therefore, the sizes of these clones are thought to range from about 1 to about 10^7 cells. However, the number of lymphocytes in the population that potentially can react with a typical antigen is much larger, because

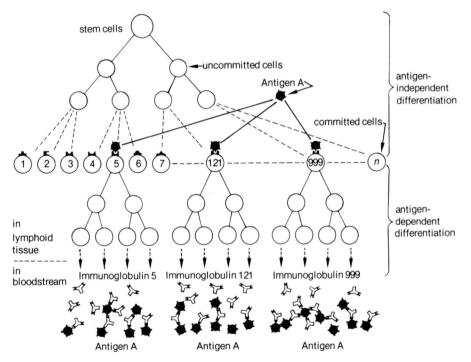

Figure 3–1 The clonal selection theory of antibody formation. Stem cell progeny undergo an antigen-independent differentiation that ultimately commits each of 10^5 to 10^8 clones to the synthesis of its own molecular species of antibody (numbers). These antibodies are displayed as receptors on the cell surfaces. A particular antigen (A) usually interacts with several clones to initiate the antigen-dependent stage of differentiation, which leads to proliferation of clones of antibody-producing cells with complementary receptors and to the synthesis of specific antibody molecules. [Adapted from G. Edelman, *Sci. Am.* **223,** 34 (1970). Copyright © 1970 by Scientific American, Inc. All rights reserved.]

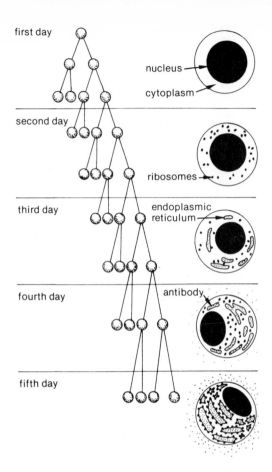

first day

nucleus

cytoplasm

second day

ribosomes

third day

endoplasmic reticulum

fourth day

antibody

fifth day

Figure 3–2 Successive stages in the development of mature plasma cells after triggering by antigen. This process, called blast transformation, takes about five days and eight cell generations. The mature plasma cell has an extensive endoplasmic reticulum whose internal cavities are filled with antibody molecules. [Adapted from G. J. V. Nossal, *Sci. Am.* **211,** 109 (1964). Copyright © 1964 by Scientific American, Inc. All rights reserved.]

such an antigen displays many determinants, and because a given determinant can be recognized by more than one kind of receptor.

C.   Lymphocytes that bind an antigen may be triggered to proliferate and differentiate in a process called *blast transformation* (Figure 3–2). They form clones of progeny lymphocytes, each of which displays surface receptors with the same antigen-binding specificity as its parent cell. In the process of proliferation, some progeny differentiate into *effector cells,* the functional end products of the immune response. The B lymphocyte effector cells are *plasma cells* (Figure 1–2b), which secrete humoral antibodies with the same antigen-binding sites as their cell-surface receptors. T lymphocytes give rise to several types of effector cells with different functions. One of these types is the *cytotoxic* or *killer T cell* (T_C cell), which eliminates foreign cells directly. Other types of effector T cells are responsible for delayed hypersensitivity (T_D cells), for helping B-cell differentiation and proliferation (T_H cells), for amplifying killer T-cell differentiation and proliferation (T_A cells), and for suppressing immune responses (T_S cells).

D.   The clonal selection process explains the phenomenon known as *immunologic memory*. For example, when a mammal first encounters an antigen, its so-called primary immune response exhibits the kinetics shown in Figure 3–3. However, if the mammal encounters the same antigen after an interval of a few days, or at any later time during its life, its specific response is more rapid and greater in magnitude. The initial encounter causes specific B- and T-cell clones to proliferate and differentiate. The progeny lymphocytes include not only effector cells, but also expanded clones of *memory cells,* which retain the capacity to produce further progeny cells of both the effector and memory types upon subsequent stimulation by the original antigen. Whereas the lifetime of an effector cell is measured in days, the memory cells produced in a primary response can remain in the lymphocyte population for decades. Thus if the same antigen is encountered again, its cognate memory cells rapidly produce large numbers of effector cells to give the rapid increases in specific humoral antibodies and effector T cells characteristic of a secondary response.

E.   The clonal selection process also must account for the phenomenon of *tolerance,* a set of mechanisms that prevents organisms from

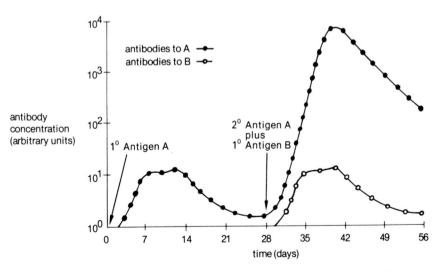

Figure 3–3 Kinetics of the appearance of immunoglobulins in the serum following primary (1⁰) and secondary (2⁰) immunizations at days 0 and 28, respectively. The secondary immunization includes a control antigen to demonstrate the specificity of immunological memory. The secondary response is both faster and greater than the primary response.

mounting immune responses to the antigenic determinants of their own macromolecules. Tolerance is induced by a process, still poorly understood, that eliminates or suppresses all clones of lymphocytes that could respond to normal constituents of the organism.

3-2   Precursor lymphocytes differentiate to produce functionally distinct T and B cells

A.   In mammals the primordial lymphocyte precursors arise in the blood islands of the yolk sac and then migrate successively to the embryonic liver and bone marrow. Throughout the remainder of the organism's lifetime the bone marrow produces blood-forming (hematopoietic) stem cells, which have lymphocyte precursors among their progeny. These cells mature through one of two developmental pathways into immunologically competent T or B cells.

B.   Maturation of both T and B cells is believed to include an antigen-independent phase and an antigen-driven phase (Figure 3-1). The differentiation steps that occur in the fetus or in organs that are not accumulating and processing foreign antigens are thought to be antigen-independent. Lymphocytes that differentiate in these environments become *immunocompetent;* that is, they acquire antigen-specific cell-surface receptors and the cellular machinery to respond to antigen stimulation. These cells are called *virgin lymphocytes.* Antigen-driven differentiation of these lymphocytes eventually results in the generation of memory cells and effector cells.

C.   Maturation of the T-cell lineage involves at least four distinct events: embryologic establishment of an appropriate microenvironment in the thymus, seeding of the thymic microenvironment by precommitted hematopoietic T-cell precursors, intrathymic proliferation and differentiation to immunocompetence, and migration to peripheral lymphoid tissues.

1.   The thymus originates embryologically with the movement of cells from one embryonic germ layer, the endoderm, into another layer, the mesoderm (mesenchyme). The third and fourth pouches of the anterior (pharyngeal) endoderm penetrate the surrounding mesenchyme to initiate formation of the thymus and parathyroids (Figure 3-4). The thymus rudiment detaches itself and migrates down into the chest cavity. For a brief interval just after its downward migration, the thymic rudiment collects T-cell precursors from the blood. Throughout life the hematopoietic tissues of the bone marrow provide a low level of thymic precursors. While in the thymus, T cells may become equipped with surface receptors for antigen and the capacity for homing to specific peripheral lymphoid T-cell domains.

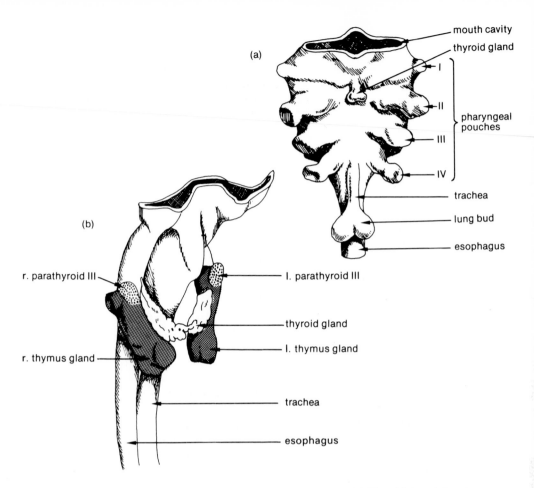

Figure 3—4 Embryological development of the thymus. (a) The third and fourth endodermal pharyngeal pouches migrate laterally into surrounding mesenchyme, and then split. The portions that remain in the neck (b) form the parathyroids, while the portions that migrate down into the chest cavity form the thymic lobes. [Adapted from G. L. Weller, *Contrib. Embryol. Carneg. Inst.* **24**, 93 (1933).]

    2. Following their migration to the periphery, the antigen-specific virgin T cells may respond to further antigenic stimulation by proliferating and terminally differentiating to memory T cells and effector T cells.

D. Maturation of B cells also involves antigen-independent induction by a microenvironment. In the process, B cells, like T cells, acquire specific homing and cell-recognition properties, as well as antigen-specific cell-surface receptor antibodies.

    1. In mammals, precommitment of hematopoietic cells to the B-cell lineage and microenvironmental induction to virgin B cells occur in the liver and perhaps in the spleen during fetal life, and in the bone marrow during adult life. Very little is known about early events in B-cell maturation, except that they include the expression of membrane-bound IgM receptor immunoglobulins.

In all vertebrate species tested, subclasses of B cells express one or both of two receptors for immunologically significant molecules: one for the Fc region of IgG immunoglobulins and the other for the activated form of a serum complement component (C3). The functional significance of these receptors is still unknown, but they provide useful markers for the identification of B cells in humans (Figure 3–5).

2.   Following their generation in bone marrow, the antigen-specific virgin B cells migrate to peripheral B-cell domains where they respond to further antigenic stimulation by proliferating and terminally differentiating to memory B cells and antibody-secreting plasma cells.

3.   In birds, development of the B-cell but not the T-cell system is prevented by exposing the embryo to the male hormone testosterone. The *bursa of Fabricius,* a lymphoid pouch that connects with the intestinal lumen, fails to develop in these birds, and B cells and plasma cells do not appear. It seems likely that the lack of a bursa and the failure of B-cell system development are linked. Many immunologists believe that the bursa is the site for generation of virgin B cells in birds; this belief gave rise to the designation "B" for bursal cells.

E.   The analysis of T- and B-cell differentiation sequences is difficult and still incomplete. Several animal and human lymphoid cancers appear to be of either T-cell or B-cell origin. Many of these cancer cell lines express different specific differentiation markers, as if frozen at various stages of maturation. For example, in humans a high proportion of acute lymphocytic leukemias bear T-cell markers, while most chronic lymphocytic leukemias bear B-cell markers.

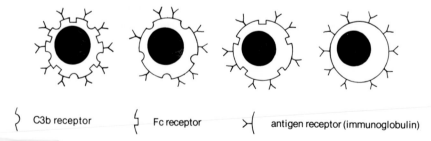

C3b receptor   Fc receptor   antigen receptor (immunoglobulin)

Figure 3–5   A diagram of four classes of B cells with differing combinations of B-cell-specific surface receptors. It is not known whether these B cells result from distinct pathways of differentiation or whether they represent different stages along a single differentiation pathway.

F.   The ontogenic maturation time of the lymphoid system relative to birth differs from one species to another. As measured by the onset of immune responsiveness as well as by the appearance of peripheral T and B cells, mice and birds develop their immune systems just before and after birth, whereas sheep and humans develop functional immune systems early in gestation, well before birth. However, in all species the immediate postnatal period is marked by dramatic differentiative changes in the immune system, reflecting the sudden exposure to a host of environmental antigens.

3-3   Lymphocytes encounter and respond to antigens in specialized lymphoid organs

A.   Lymphocytes are carried throughout most of the tissues and organs of higher vertebrates by two circulatory networks, the blood and lymphatic systems. Lymphocytes make up 20–80% of the nucleated cells in the blood, and over 99% of the nucleated cells in the lymphatic fluid (lymph). However, lymphocytes contact and respond to immunizing antigens in specialized lymphoid organs that provide accessory cells and tissue architecture appropriate for antigen processing and presentation. The lymphoid system (Figure 3–6) has three principal functions: (1) to concentrate antigens from all parts of the body into a few lymphoid organs; (2) to circulate the lymphocyte population through these organs, so that every antigen is exposed to a representation of the organism's repertoire of antigen-specific lymphocytes in a short period of time; and (3) to carry the products of the immune response, antigen-specific effector T cells and humoral antibodies, to the bloodstream and the tissues.

B.   Antigens are collected and processed by different lymphoid organs, depending upon their route of entry into the body. Processing in all these organs involves white blood cells called *phagocytes* (*phago*, eating; *cyte*, cell), which take up antigens from the circulating fluid for presentation to lymphocytes. The large phagocytes found in lymphoid organs are called *macrophages*.

1.   Antigens that enter the intercellular spaces of any tissue are swept into the lymph nodes of the lymphatic system. Lymphatic vessels originate in the interstitial spaces of the tissues. Interstitial lymph fluid is pulled into and pumped through the lymphatics by osmotic pressure and muscular contraction. The fluid is transported through *afferent lymphatic* vessels to lymph nodes. It enters a node through a series of cavities (*sinusoids*) that are lined with macrophages, and percolates through the tissue of the lymph node.

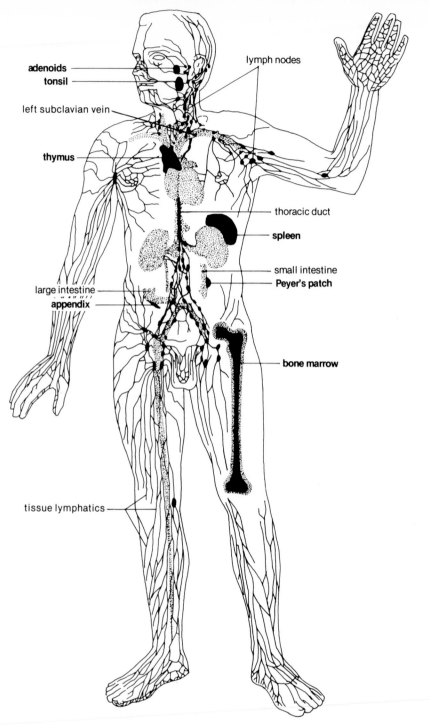

Figure 3–6 A diagram of the human lymphoid system. The system consists of circulating lymphocytes and the lymphatic organs, which include the tree of lymphatic vessels and the lymph nodes stationed along them, the bone marrow (in the long bones, only one of which is illustrated), the thymus, the spleen, the adenoids, the tonsils, the Peyer's patches of the small intestine, and the appendix. The lymphatic vessels collect the lymphocytes and antibody molecules from the tissues and lymph nodes and return them to the bloodstream at the subclavian veins. [Adapted from N. K. Jerne, *Sci. Am.* **229,** 52 (1973). Copyright © 1973 by Scientific American, Inc. All rights reserved.]

The typical lymph node (Figure 3–7) is a bean-shaped organ that consists of an outer layer, the *cortex*, and an inner core called the *medulla*. A fibrous tissue network (reticulum) throughout the node supports macrophages and extensively branched *dendritic reticular cells;* the reticulum and its adherent cells trap antigens and provide passageways and niches for lymphocytes and their progeny (Figure 3–8).

Lymph fluid exits from the lymph node via an *efferent lymphatic* vessel. Several efferent lymphatics come together and fuse into larger lymphatic ducts, which in turn empty into the venous system.

2. Antigens that enter the body via the upper respiratory and gastrointestinal tracts are filtered through local lymph nodes as well as through several specialized lymphoid organs: the tonsils, adenoids, Peyer's patches, and appendix (Figure 3–6).

3. Antigens that enter the bloodstream are filtered out by macrophages that line sinusoidal blood vessels in the spleen, liver, and lungs. However, only the spleen is capable of mounting

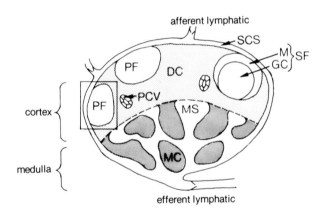

Figure 3–7   The general structure of a lymph node. The cortical subcapsular sinus (SCS) lies beneath the capsule of the node and communicates extensively with the sinuses of the medulla. The subcapsular sinus drains the extracellular space via afferent lymphatics, and is lined with phagocytic cells. The primary follicle (PF), lying directly under the SCS in the cortex, is an ovoid accumulation of small lymphocytes lying in a meshwork of dendritic reticular cells. The secondary follicle (SF) is composed of the mantle (M), the components of which are similar to those of the primary follicle, and the germinal center (GC), which contains small and large lymphocytes, many large blast cells with abundant cytoplasm, "tingible body" macrophages (containing phagocytized cell debris), and dendritic reticular cells. The diffuse cortex (DC) includes many small lymphocytes, macrophages, and postcapillary venules (PCV). The medullary sinus (MS) is lined by phagocytic cells. This sinus constitutes the route of emigration of itinerant T and B lymphocytes, as well as blast cells after antigen stimulation. The medullary cords (MC) are close-packed, interconnected spaces containing cords of cells, particularly plasma cells and large lymphoblasts.

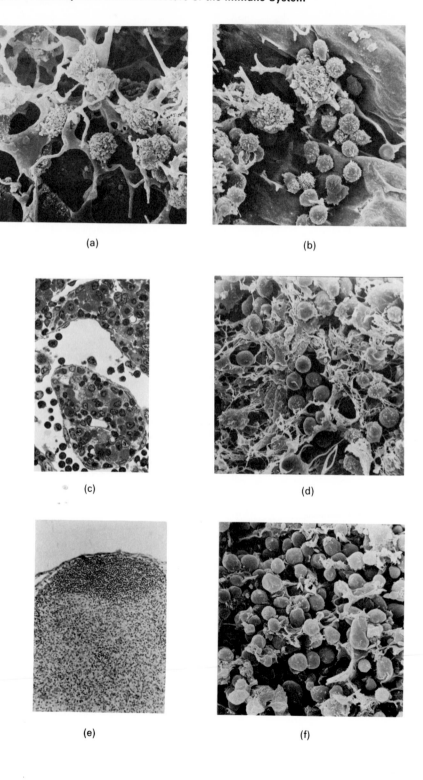

(a)

(b)

(c)

(d)

(e)

(f)

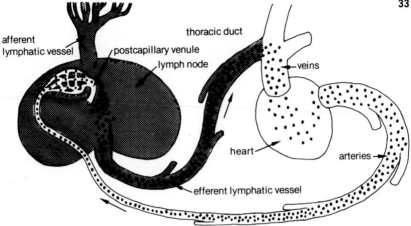

Figure 3–9 The pathway of lymphocyte recirculation. Blood lymphocytes enter lymph nodes, adhere to the walls of specialized postcapillary venules, and migrate to the lymph node diffuse cortex. Many lymphocytes then migrate to T- or B-cell domains and percolate through lymphoid fields to medullary lymphatic sinuses and then to efferent lymphatics, which in turn collect into major lymphatic ducts in the thorax that empty into the neck veins leading to the heart. [Redrawn from J. Gowans, *Hosp. Pract.* **3(3),** 34 (1968).]

an immune response to blood-borne antigens. The spleen is differentiated into two types of tissue, called *lymphoid white pulp* and *erythroid red pulp.* The white pulp is analogous in structure and function to the cortex of the lymph node. The red pulp is involved in scavenging old red blood cells (*erythrocytes*), and is a reserve site for hematopoiesis.

C.   Recirculating lymphocytes pass from the blood through the lymphoid system and back to the blood. On the way they percolate through lymphoid organs where they may contact processed antigens (Figure 3–9).

← **Figure 3–8**   Microscopic anatomy of a lymph node. (a) Scanning electron micrograph (SEM) of the subcapsular sinus; the flattened bodies with long branching processes are part of the reticulum, and the adherent cells with multiple globular protrusions are macrophages. Notice the large intercellular spaces in the sinus. (b) SEM of the medullary sinus; again a flattened reticulum with adherent macrophages is evident. The smaller round cells with or without filamentous protrusions are lymphocytes, and a biconcave red blood cell is seen at the right. (c) An electron microscopic view of a cross-section of the medulla. The clear space is the medullary sinus with a few large pale macrophages and many small dark lymphocytes. The highly cellular portions are medullary cords, containing lymphoblasts and plasma cells. (d) SEM view of the diffuse cortex, where a fine meshwork of reticulum surrounds many lymphocytes. (e) Light microscopic view of a standard histological section of a lymph node from a thymus-deprived mouse. The only region containing large numbers of small, dark, round lymphocytes is the primary follicle. (f) SEM view of a primary follicle; dendritic reticular cells with long lacy processes surround densely-packed small lymphocytes. [Electron micrographs (a)–(d) and (f) courtesy of W. van Ewijk; (e) photomicrograph by I. Weissman.]

(a)

(b)

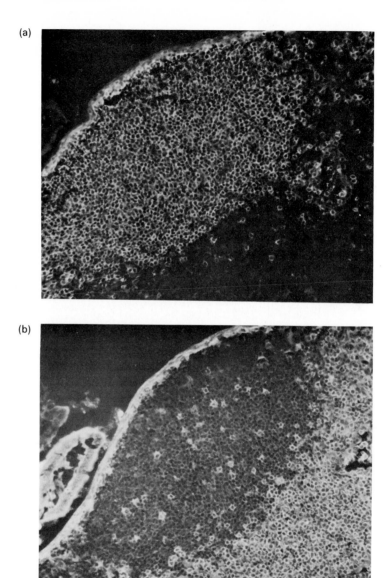

Figure 3–10   Localization of T and B cells in a lymph node. A lymph node was frozen rapidly, and sections of the node were stained with antibodies coupled to a fluorescent tracer. Photomicrographs were taken to locate bound fluorescent antibodies.(a) Anti-B-cell fluorescent antibodies were used to stain the cortex of a node containing a primary follicle (top left) and its adjacent diffuse cortex (bottom right) containing a postcapillary venule (PCV). B cells predominate in the primary follicle; they are found also in the lumen and wall of the PCV, presumably just having entered via the bloodstream. (b) A serial section adjacent to the one in (a), stained with anti-T-cell fluorescent antibodies. T cells predominate in the diffuse cortex and also are found in the PCV. [Photomicrographs by G. A. Gutman and I. Weissman.]

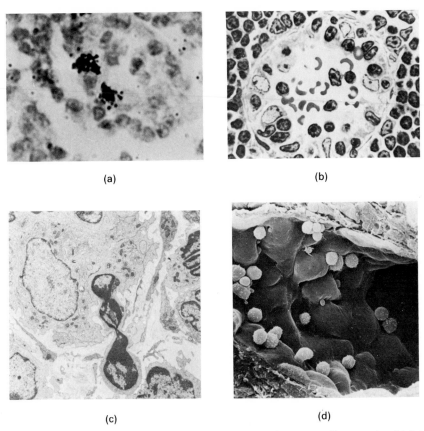

(a)

(b)

(c)

(d)

Figure 3–11 Microscopic views of lymphocytes traversing postcapillary venules. (a) An autoradiograph of labeled lymphocytes in the walls of a postcapillary venule within minutes after their injection into the bloodstream [G. A. Gutman and I. Weissman, *Transplantation* **16**, 621 (1973)]. (b) A thin section of a postcapillary venule under high power, showing lymphocytes in different stages of passage with several red blood cells in the vessel lumen. [Photomicrograph courtesy of G. Levine.] (c) An electron microscopic view of a lymphocyte (lower right) squeezing through a narrow passageway in a postcapillary venule. Lymphocyte nuclei stain densely, while endothelial nuclei stain lightly with a dark rim just inside the nuclear membrane. [Electron micrograph courtesy of G. Levine and G. A. Gutman.] (d) A scanning electron microscopic view of several lymphocytes in contact with the inner surface of postcapillary venule endothelial cells. [Electron micrograph courtesy of W. van Ewijk.]

1. In the resting lymph node the cortex is divided into discrete B-cell domains, called the *primary follicles*, and an adjacent T-cell domain, the *diffuse cortex* (Figures 3–7 and 3–10). Lymphocytes enter the lymph node from the bloodstream via arterioles and capillaries to reach postcapillary venules in the diffuse cortex. Both T and B cells, but not other blood cells, adhere specifically to large, specialized endothelial cells in the venule walls, and then traverse these walls to enter the node (Figure 3–11). Upon entry, B cells migrate to the follicles and T cells remain in the diffuse cortex.

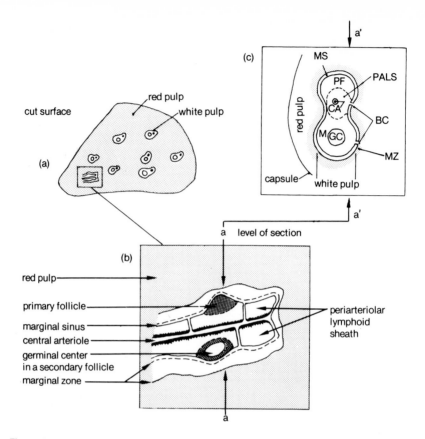

Figure 3–12 General structure of a spleen. (a) A cross-section of the spleen. (b) Enlargement of an area of white pulp. (c) Cross-section of an area of white pulp. *White pulp:* The central arteriole (CA), a branch of a trabecular artery, has branches that empty into the marginal zone (MZ), marginal sinus (MS), and red pulp. The periarteriolar lymphoid sheath (PALS) is an accumulation of small lymphocytes surrounding the central arteriole. The primary follicles (PF), mantle (M), and germinal center (GC) are similar to those described for the lymph node (Figure 3–7). *Marginal area:* The marginal sinus (MS) separates the white pulp from the marginal zone (MZ) and red pulp. The marginal areas, including the sinuses, receive much of the blood entering the spleen. These areas are major sites of entry of T and B cells. Bridging channels (BC) appear to interrupt the marginal area and form connections between the white and red pulp. *Red pulp:* In addition to hematopoietic cells (in the mouse), plasma cells appear in this site and are particularly prominent after antigenic stimulation.

In resting lymph nodes, the medulla serves primarily as a collecting point for sinusoids that lead to the efferent lymphatic vessels. After traversing their specific cortical domains, recirculating B and T cells enter these sinusoids, and then are transported via the main lymphatic ducts back into the venous system for recirculation. The lymphocyte fields of the lymph nodes thus contain slowly moving masses of B and T cells, most of which are on their way from blood to lymph and back to blood.

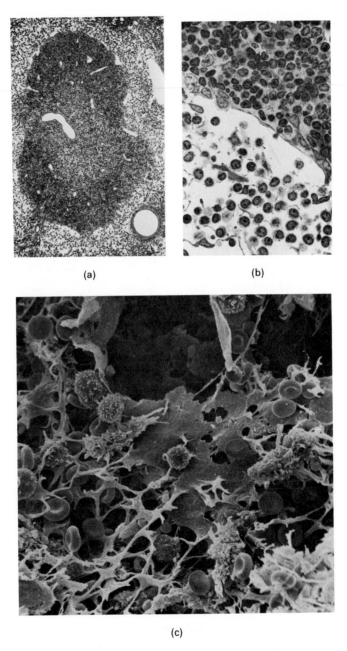

(a) (b)

(c)

Figure 3–13 Microscopic anatomy of the spleen. (a) A light micrograph of a section of the spleen. The structures have the same relationship to each other as diagramed in Figure 3–12c. (b) An electron microscopic view of a primary follicle (upper right) and the marginal zone (lower left). One cell appears to be traversing the boundary. (c) A scanning electron microscopic view of the marginal zone. The dendritic reticulum and its adherent macrophages surround the space containing lymphocytes and red blood cells. [Electron micrographs courtesy of W. van Ewijk.]

(a)

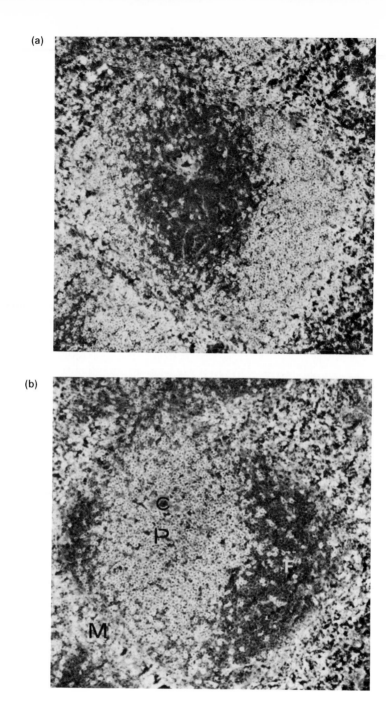

(b)

Figure 3–14 Localization of T and B cells in the spleen. Photomicrographs are of sections stained as in Figure 3–10. (a) Anti-B-cell stain of a spleen. The central arteriole (C) is immediately surrounded by a fluorescent-negative periarteriolar lymphoid sheath (P). B cells predominate in the eccentric follicles (F) and are interspersed around the marginal zone (M). (b) Anti-T-cell stain of serial section: T cells predominate in the periarteriolar lymphoid sheath and are interspersed around the marginal zone. [Micrographs by G. A. Gutman and I. Weissman.]

2. Most lymphocytes enter and leave the spleen directly via the bloodstream. The lymphoid white pulp of the spleen (Figure 3–12) takes the form of a bumpy sheath that surrounds entering arterioles. It is separated from the red pulp by the marginal zone, which receives blood from a specialized venule called the marginal sinus. This sinus arises at the termination of the arteriole and curves back to envelop the white pulp. The bumps on the sheath are primary follicles, that is, B-cell domains, whereas the sheath itself consists of T-cell domains (Figures 3–13 and 3–14). Circulating B and T cells, but no other blood cells, enter the white pulp by traversing the walls of the marginal sinus, and then migrate to their respective domains. Lymphocytes then leave the spleen either via splenic veins or via splenic efferent lymphatics.

Thus in the absence of antigenic stimulation lymphocytes recirculate from blood to lymphoid organs and eventually back to blood via the large lymphatic trunks. In the blood and lymphatic vessels, these T and B lymphocytes are intermixed, whereas within lymphoid organs they are segregated from each other. Antigenic stimulation activates cognate lymphocyte clones, altering the morphology of both the cells and the lymphoid organs. The subsequent immune response is the subject of Chapter 4.

Selected Bibliography

Burnet, F. M., "A modification of Jerne's theory of antibody production using the concept of clonal selection," *Aust. J. Sci.* **20**, 67 (1957). The theoretical basis for modern immunology. This article clearly defines the basic unit of selection as cells, not molecules.

Gowans, J. L., McGregor, D. D., Cowen, D. M., and Ford, C. E., "Initiation of immune responses by small lymphocytes," *Nature* **196**, 651 (1962). Proof that the cellular units of selection in the immune response are lymphocytes.

Raff, M. C., "Cell-surface immunology," *Sci. Am.* **234**, 30 (1976).

Weissman, I. L., Gutman, G. A., and Friedberg, S. H., "Tissue localization of lymphoid cells," *Ser. Haematol.* **8**, 482 (1974). The organization of lymphocytes in the lymphoid system is detailed in this review.

Exercises

3–1   Indicate whether each of the following statements is true or false. Explain the error in each statement you consider to be false.

T (a)   T cells are derived from hematopoietic stem cells.

F (b)   B cells that enter the spleen, home to the lymphoid white pulp of the periarteriolar sheath.

T (c)   A lymphocyte is generally committed to express one type of antibody molecule.

T (d)   Plasma cells, killer T cells, and suppressor T cells are examples of effector cells.

F (e)   B cells mature in the thymus.

T (f)   Antigens that enter interstitial spaces in any tissue are transported to lymph nodes via the lymphatic system.

T (g)   Antigens that enter the bloodstream are filtered out by macrophages in the spleen.

F (h)   The primary follicles of lymph nodes are T-cell domains.

3–2   Supply the missing word or words in each of the following statements.

(a)   The clonal selection theory contends that lymphocytes commit themselves to the synthesis of one type of antibody molecule prior to exposure to _antigen_, but that _antigen_ triggers the final stage of differentiation, called blast transformation.

(b)   Accessory cells involved in antigen processing include _macrophages_ and _dendritic, reticular cells_

(c)   _Killer_ or _cytotoxic_ T cells are effector cells that eliminate foreign cells directly.

(d)   _Tolerance_ is a set of mechanisms that prevent organisms from mounting immune responses to their own macromolecules.

(e)   _Virgin_ lymphocytes have never been exposed to antigen.

(f)   In the spleen, B-cell and T-cell domains both are found in the _white pulp_.

(g)   A lymph node is supplied with lymph fluid by the _afferent_ lymphatic vessels.

(h)   In a lymph node antigen is trapped by _macrophages_ and _dendritic, reticular cells_

(i)   Most chronic lymphocytic leukemias are of the _B_ cell type.

(j)   Many immunologists believe that in birds, the _bursa_ is the site of B-cell maturation.

(k)   Once a lymphocyte can respond to antigen, it is said to be _immunocompetent_

Answers are given on page 155.

4 THE IMMUNE RESPONSE

The delivery of antigen to lymphoid organs triggers into action one of the most complex systems in the vertebrate organism. The antigen first is processed to achieve the most efficient presentation of its antigenic determinants to T and B lymphocytes. These lymphocytes interact with each other, proliferate to enlarge their clones, and differentiate to effector cells. Effector cells and their products then combine with antigen and induce several other serum factors and cells to aid in elimination responses. The system is regulated at several levels, in order to prevent any responses against self, and in order to coordinate activation and deactivation of the immune response according to the magnitude of the antigenic load. This chapter considers the cellular and molecular biology of the vertebrate immune response.

Essential Concepts

4-1 Antigen binding to lymphocyte surface receptors triggers an immune response

A. Antigen-triggered lymphocyte proliferation and differentiation occurs in lymphoid organs. Within minutes after infection or injection, antigen enters lymph nodes via the afferent lymphatics and is taken up by macrophages. Most of this antigen becomes incorporated into special vacuoles, called *phagosomes,* in the cytoplasm of macrophages. The vacuoles fuse with *lysosomes,* vesicles that contain hydrolytic enzymes, to form *phagolysosomes.* The enzymes degrade most of the antigen to nonantigenic components. However, the macrophage cell surface retains or receives a small amount of highly immunogenic material for presentation to antigen-specific lymphocytes.

B. Binding of a cognate antigen to the surface receptors of either T or B lymphocytes, triggers a general activation, called *blast transformation* (Figures 3–2 and 4–1). The activated cells proliferate and differentiate, with concomitant changes in the morphology of the lymph node.

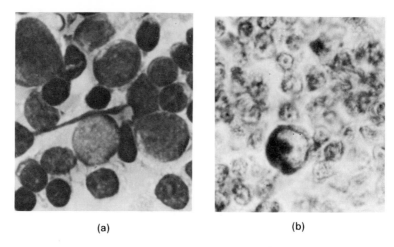

(a)   (b)

Figure 4–1   Antigen-induced activation of T cells. (a) The appearance of a T cell (lymphoblast) activated *in vitro* and surrounded by resting T cells. (b) The appearance of an activated T cell in the tissue. The peculiar morphology of this cell is emphasized by using a dye (pyronin Y), which stains RNA intensely. [Photographs courtesy of R. Rouse.]

During the first 24–48 hours following antigenic stimulation of the organism, antigen-specific lymphocyte clones are retained in lymphoid organs that contain the antigen. During this period these clones are largely depleted from the recirculating lymphocyte population.

1.   A focus of dividing T and B cells as well as active macrophages builds up in the follicle to form a *germinal center,* which compresses the follicle into a crescent around it. Follicles that contain germinal centers, known as secondary follicles (Figure 4–2), appear 4–5 days after antigen injection, and may remain for several days. At the same time plasma cells begin to settle between the sinusoids of the medulla, to form medullary cords. Other activated B-cell progeny, as well as most activated T cells and their progeny, percolate through the lymph node and spread to other lymphoid tissues and the bloodstream via the efferent lymphatics and the major lymphatic ducts. Thus most memory and effector T cells and memory B cells eventually reenter the general circulation following antigenic stimulation, whereas most plasma cells are retained in the lymph node.

2.   Following antigenic stimulation of a lymph node, activated B and T cells release soluble factors that cause local vessel dilation, which allows leakage (transudation) of plasma fluids into the lymph node. Other factors may attract macrophages and other blood phagocytes into the node. The resulting accumulation of cells and fluid may plug some of the medullary

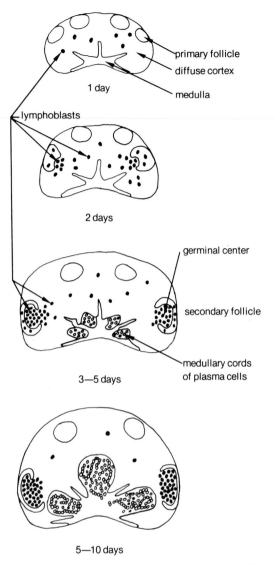

Figure 4–2 Morphological changes in a lymph node after stimulation with a thymus-dependent antigen. The diagram depicts the time course of antigen-dependent changes in multi-cellular structures, and emphasizes changes in size and shape of the separate lymphoid compartments, largely caused by selective proliferation and altered movement patterns of lymphocyte subclasses. Analogous changes occur in antigen-activated spleen.

sinusoids that lead to efferent lymphatics. The combination of specific cellular proliferation, increased fluid in the tissues (edema), increased numbers of nonlymphoid cells, and retention of normally recirculating lymphocytes causes the lymph node to enlarge rapidly. This enlargement causes typical "swollen glands" of infection, which return to their original size only as the response to infection abates.

C.   The products of an immune response in any lymphoid tissue are effector T cells and humoral antibodies produced by plasma cells. These products, which must be distributed to the bloodstream and the tissues to play their defensive roles, are transported via efferent lymphatic vessels and lymphatic ducts into the venous system. Of the five classes of humoral antibodies, IgG can traverse blood vessel walls and enter the interstitial spaces of tissues most efficiently. Typically about 50% of an organism's IgG antibodies are found in the interstitial fluid and 50% in the bloodstream. The remaining classes of circulating antibodies, IgA, IgD, IgE, and IgM, are confined primarily to the bloodstream or to specific local sites.

Effector T cells in the bloodstream collect rapidly on blood-vessel walls near a site where cognate antigens have invaded the tissues. The T cells then migrate through the vessel walls into the tissues, where they initiate inflammatory and elimination responses to the invading agent.

4-2   The antibodies produced in a humoral immune response are heterogeneous in specificity and may include all immunoglobulin classes

A.   An individual B cell activated by a cognate antigen proliferates and differentiates to form plasma cells, which begin to synthesize identical antibodies with a single specificity at the rate of 3,000 to 30,000 molecules per cell per second. However, an organism's total response to the simplest antigens almost always is heterogeneous with respect to antibody specificity. This heterogeneity is due to two factors: most antigens have multiple antigenic determinants that trigger the activation of different B cells, and even a single antigenic determinant generally activates several different B cells that display receptor immunoglobulins with similar but not identical specificities (Figure 4–3). Consequently the serum of any vertebrate contains an extremely heterogeneous collection of immunoglobulin molecules whose specificities reflect the organism's past antigenic history.

B.   The B-cell response to a single antigen may produce antibody molecules of all five known classes of immunoglobulins: IgA, IgD, IgE, IgG, and IgM. Antibodies of the five classes mediate different physiological effector functions (Table 4–1). They are present in normal human serum at very different concentrations, and they differ significantly in normal serum half-life. In addition, the five classes are produced in different relative amounts in primary and secondary immune responses (Figure 4–4).

1.   IgM, the first antibody produced in response to an immunogen, is a pentamer of the basic antibody structural unit. IgM

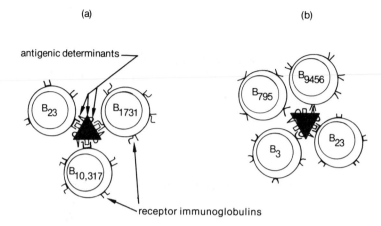

Figure 4–3 Two sources of heterogeneity in an antibody response to an antigen. (a) The same antigenic determinant triggers B cells with functionally related but different receptor immunoglobulins. (b) Different antigenic determinants on the same antigen trigger B cells with different receptors.

Table 4–1

Physiological properties of the five immunoglobulin classes in humans

Class	Mean adult serum level (mg/ml)	Serum half-life (days)	Physiological functions
IgM	1.0	5	Complement fixation; early immune response; stimulation of ingestion by macrophages
IgG	12	25	Complement fixation; placental transfer; stimulation of ingestion by macrophages
IgA	1.8	6	Localized protection in external secretions
IgD	0.03	2.8	Function unknown
IgE	0.0003	2	Stimulation of mast cells; possibly parasite expulsion

is particularly effective against invading microorganisms. Although the affinity of each IgM active site for a cognate antigenic determinant may be low, the overall avidity of the IgM pentamer for a complex antigen is very high, due to the presence of repeating determinants on most complex cell-membrane antigens. Because of its pentameric structure, IgM, on a molar basis, is many-fold

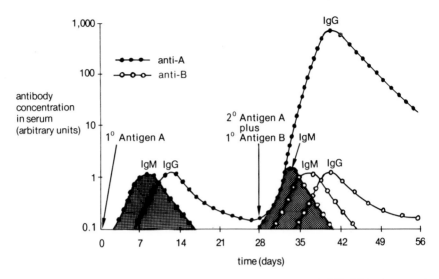

Figure 4–4   Kinetics of IgM and IgG appearance in the serum following primary and secondary immunizations. The secondary response to Antigen A demonstrates that the IgM response is slightly more rapid and intense than the primary IgG response. However, most of the secondary response is of the IgG class.

times more effective at agglutinating cells by cross-linking than are monomeric divalent antibodies. In addition, IgM bound to an antigenic target cell stimulates its ingestion by macrophages and its destruction by complement fixation (Essential Concept 4–3).

IgM is principally an antibody of the blood. Because of its large size it enters the interstitial fluid slowly, if at all. It does not cross the placenta to enter the fetal circulation. IgM also is displayed as a monomer on the surfaces of B cells, where it may act as a receptor immunoglobulin.

2.   IgG is a monomeric antibody produced later in the immune response than IgM. IgG is the most prevalent antibody in the blood, and is a major antibody in tissue spaces. The prevalence of IgG in the bloodstream makes it a major trigger of complement fixation, although on a molar basis it is many times less effective than IgM at this function. IgG also activates macrophage ingestion of antigenic particles by coating them with antibody. IgG is the only class of antibody that can cross the placenta to provide immunity for a developing fetus.

3.   IgA, also produced later in an immune response than IgM, can exist as a monomer, dimer, or trimer of the basic immunoglobulin structural unit. IgA antibodies are thought to act as a

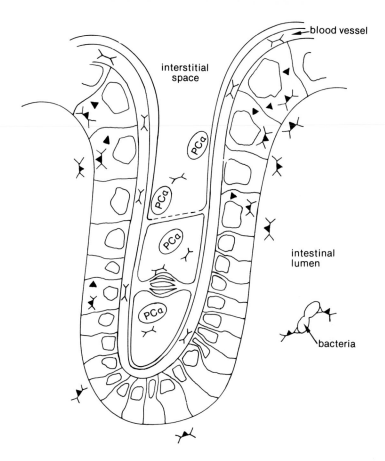

Figure 4–5 Representation of intestinal villus with epithelial cells producing secretory component (▲), which facilitates the transport of dimeric IgA (>—<) from the interstitial spaces into the intestinal lumen. PC$_\alpha$ indicates IgA-producing plasma cells in the interstitial space of the villus.

protective barrier against microorganisms at several potential points of entry. Some epithelial cells produce a polypeptide called secretory component (Sc), which complexes to the Fc region of IgA antibodies and specifically mediates their transport from interstitial spaces to the epithelial surface (Figure 4–5).

B-cell precursors of IgA-secreting plasma cells are found in highest frequency in lymphoid organs that drain the gastrointestinal tract. Upon antigenic stimulation, progeny of these lymphocytes are released into the bloodstream via efferent lymphatics and collecting ducts. Most of these cells home preferentially to the gastrointestinal tract, where they come to rest in the tissue spaces just under the epithelial mucosal cells, and there differentiate to IgA-secreting plasma cells.

Similar precursor lymphocytes home to the mammary gland, where they differentiate into IgA-secreting plasma cells just under the epithelial glandular cells. IgA is a major immunoglobulin in milk and colostrum, where it may function to protect the gastrointestinal tracts of nursing infants. IgA also is found in saliva, tears, and sweat.

4.   IgD, a monomeric antibody, normally is present in only minute concentrations in the blood. It also is present as a cell-surface receptor on a majority of circulating B cells, but its functions are still unknown.

5.   IgE, a monomeric, heat-labile antibody, also is normally present in the blood in only minute concentrations. IgE antibodies bind tightly via their Fc regions to *mast cells* in connective tissue and to blood basophiles. Interaction of bound IgE with a cognate antigen can trigger the mast cell to *degranulate*, that is, to release the contents of its intracellular vacuoles, which contain *histamine* and a sulfated polysaccharide called *heparin* (Figure 4–6). The release of histamine results in local vessel dilation and smooth muscle contraction.

C.   A given plasma cell secretes antibody of only one class. The class that a plasma cell secretes generally is the same as the class of receptor immunoglobulin displayed by its B-cell precursor. Mature B cells and memory B cells that display the various classes of immunoglobulins as receptors are designated by the corresponding Greek letters: for example, B_μ cells carry monomeric IgM molecules as receptors, B_γ cells carry IgG molecules as receptors, and so on. Plasma cells are designated in the same manner, as PC_μ, PC_γ, and so on.

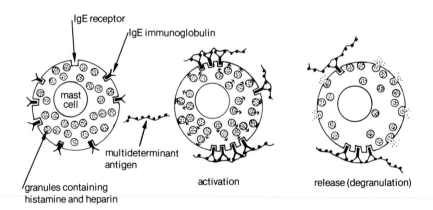

Figure 4–6   Activation of a mast cell by multivalent antigen bound to passively acquired IgE. Activation leads to the exocytosis of granules containing heparin and histamine, and to their release into the extracellular fluid.

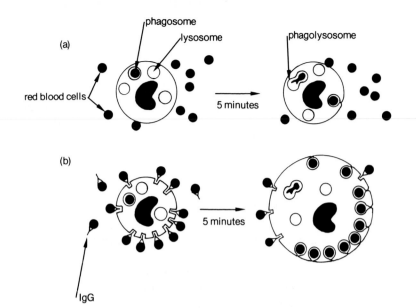

Figure 4–7 Macrophage phagocytosis of red blood cells (RBC) in the absence (a) or presence (b) of antibodies. Antibody (IgG) bound to RBC's allows macrophages with receptors for the Fc portion of the IgG molecules to bind them to the macrophage surface. Because each RBC is coated with many antibodies, the macrophage–Fc bond to any one RBC is multivalent. Bound RBC's are engulfed by membrane–Fc interactions that continue over the entire RBC surface, until macrophage membranes meet and fuse. The resulting intracellular vesicle that contains the RBC is called a phagosome. This vesicle fuses with a lysosome, and lysosome enzymes digest the RBC. Opsonizing antibody increases the number of RBC's bound to the macrophage membrane, but does not increase the rate of phagocytosis (per RBC) and digestion.

4-3   Humoral antibodies initiate several effector mechanisms for eliminating foreign cells and macromolecules

A. The biological activity of some foreign invaders is neutralized by simple combination with antibody of any class. For example, the binding of antibodies to toxins or destructive foreign enzymes, such as snake venom esterases, inhibits the interaction of these macromolecules with target ligands or substrates. Binding of antibody to surface components of viruses can prevent their attachment to target cells. Thus the humoral antibody response is effective in combating the extracellular phase of a viral infection.

B. Prior to an antibody response, the phagocytic cells of the blood—monocytes, macrophages, and polymorphonuclear leukocytes (PMN's; Figure 1–2f)—bind and ingest foreign substances. However, the rate of binding and phagocytosis increases by an order of magnitude if the foreign substance is coated with IgG antibodies. This process of preparing foreign particles for ingestion by phagocytes is called *opsonization*, and the specifically bound antibodies are called *opsonins* (Figure 4–7). Phagocytic cells bear multiple low-affinity receptors for

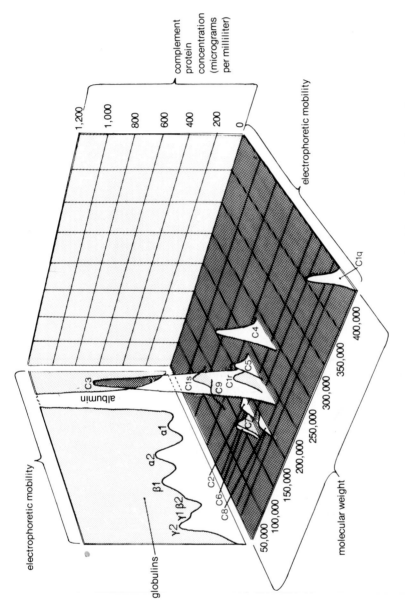

Figure 4–8 Human complement proteins characterized by molecular weights, electrophoretic mobilities at pH 8.6, and concentrations in the blood serum. For purposes of comparison, the mobilities and concentrations of globulins (α, β, and γ) and albumin are shown as well. [From M. Mayer, "The Complement System," *Sci. Am.* **229**, 54 (1973). Copyright © 1973 by Scientific American, Inc. All rights reserved.]

the constant regions of IgG molecules. A particle coated with many IgG molecules binds with high avidity to these receptors and triggers phagocytosis.

   1. Cells in the monocyte lineage may interact with IgG-coated foreign cells to cause contact lysis rather than phagocytosis. This process, called antibody-dependent cell-mediated cytotoxicity (ADCC), is independent of the complement system (defined in the following section). The effector cells for this process, called killer (K) cells, are distinct from the cytotoxic killer T cells, and are mainly nonphagocytic members of the monocyte-macrophage lineage. Thus cells of this lineage are important both in initiating and effecting immune responses.

   2. Another recently recognized type of killer cell is active against the transformed cells of virus-induced leukemias. This so-called natural killer (NK) cell does not bear T-cell or B-cell differentiation markers. Its relationship to the K cell of the monocyte-macrophage lineage is unknown.

C.   IgM and most subclasses of IgG antibodies activate the *complement system* when they bind to foreign antigens. The complement system is a set of eleven proteins that constitute about 10% of the globulins in the normal serum of man and other vertebrates (Figure 4–8). Complement proteins are distinct from immunoglobulins. The complement system is triggered by antigen–antibody complexes to initiate a cascade of proteolytic cleavage and protein-binding reactions, with at least three important consequences for host defense (Figure 4–9). First, if the antigen–antibody complex is on the surface of a foreign cell, activated complement components attack the cell membrane to cause lysis and cell death. The utilization of complement components in this process is called *complement fixation.* Second, a cleavage product of complement component C3 binds to foreign particles that have complexed with antibodies. The attached C3 fragment (C3b) interacts with C3b-specific receptors on phagocytic cells to promote the process of immune adherence, which is similar to opsonization. Third, release of other cleavage products results in the development of a local, acute inflammatory reaction that walls off the area and attracts large numbers of phagocytic polymorphonuclear leukocytes.

   Upon binding of the final complement components, C8 and C9, the cell membrane develops characteristic circular lesions (Figure 4–10) that permit cell contents to leak out. Since no concomitant covalent changes in the membrane constituents have been detected, the lesions probably do not result from direct enzymatic attack.

   An alternative pathway of complement activation is important in host defense against gram-negative bacteria that inhabit the gastrointestinal tract. Lipopolysaccharides (endotoxins) from the cell walls of

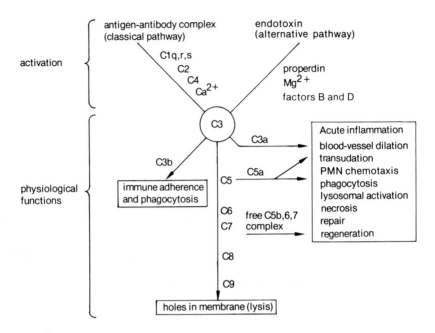

Figure 4–9   Activation pathways and physiological functions of complement components.

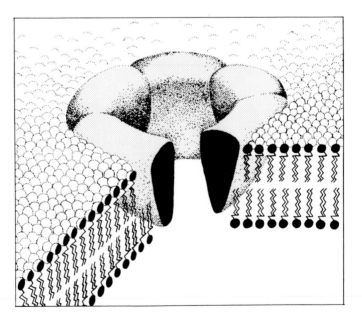

Figure 4–10 Hypothetical model of a cell-membrane pore created by a complement action. [Adapted from M. Mayer, "The Complement System," *Sci. Am.* **229,** 54 (1973). Copyright © 1973 by Scientific American, Inc. All rights reserved.

these organisms combine directly with a serum factor called *properdin,* which then, in the presence of Mg^{2+} and two serum cofactors designated D and B, cleaves C3 as in the "classical" pathway. This alternative pathway bypasses the need for antibody, C1, C4, or C2, and thus allows the complement system to be activated acutely in response to some infections.

D.   Inflammation, a common host response to injury, can be induced by antigen–antibody reactions that activate the complement system. The four cardinal signs of inflammation are *heat* (calor), *redness* (rubor), *swelling* (tumor), and *pain* (dolor).

1.   *Acute* inflammatory responses, induced by antibodies or other agents, involve a rapid set of events at the site of injury (Figure 4–11a). Local vessel dilation (which causes redness and heat) allows influx of plasma proteins and phagocytic cells into the tissue spaces (to cause swelling). Local release or activation of other vessel-active enzymes, and increased tissue pressure, trigger local nerve endings (to cause pain).

If the acute response rids the host of the agents that induce inflammation, repair and regeneration ensue. If not, the continued influx of polymorphonuclear leukocytes and serum products leads to cell death and, in some cases, to the formation of an abcess—a swelling bounded by fibrin from clotted blood and cells involved in phagocytosis and repair, with a central cavity of live and dead polymorphonuclear leukocytes, tissue debris, and the injurious or infectious agents. The center of an abcess is said to be purulent, and the liquid it contains is commonly known as pus.

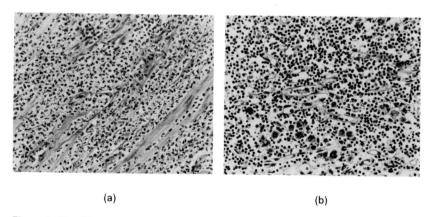

(a)   (b)

Figure 4–11   Photomicrographs of (a) acute and (b) chronic inflammation. Polymorphonuclear leukocytes predominate in acute inflammation, whereas lymphocytes and macrophages predominate in chronic inflammation. [Photomicrographs by R. Rouse and I. Weissman.]

2. Continuing acute inflammatory responses may become chronic inflammatory responses, with the same four cardinal signs, but different cellular and soluble-protein participants. Chronic inflammatory responses are characterized by an infiltration of lymphocytes and cells of the monocyte–macrophage lineage (Figure 4–11b). These responses may be induced by immunological injury initiated by effector T cells.

3. Both acute (antibody-induced) and chronic (T-cell induced) inflammation may occur in the skin. These responses are called *immediate* and *delayed hypersensitivity*, respectively. Immediate hypersensitivity, which is mediated by complement activation, begins within hours of antibody-induced immunological injury, usually peaks in intensity by 24 hours, and subsides by 48 hours. A special case of immediate hypersensitivity, induced by antigen, IgE, and mast cells, and *not* mediated by complement, arises within minutes of antigen–IgE binding, subsiding several hours later. Delayed hypersensitivity first becomes apparent 1–2 days after T-cell-induced immunological injury, peaking in intensity at 48–72 hours, and subsiding thereafter.

E.   IgE antibodies on the surfaces of mast cells bind antigens from multicellular parasites and initiate mast-cell degranulation. As a result, histamine and heparin are released, thereby causing vasodilation and smooth-muscle contraction. Although the full functional significance of the IgE system is still a mystery, it is believed that this process promotes the expulsion of parasites from organs that are surrounded with smooth muscle, such as the gastrointestinal tract and uterus. Blood IgE levels rise significantly in individuals with gastrointestinal parasites such as worms and helminths. These individuals have high concentrations of intestinal mast cells coated with IgE. Blood IgE levels also are high in allergic individuals.

4–4   Effector T cells cooperate with B cells to produce a humoral immune response

A.   Antibody molecules are synthesized only by the progeny of B cells. However, certain effector T cells serve to facilitate the differentiation of B cells into plasma cells. Cooperation between B and T cells requires an antigen that carries at least two different antigenic determinants, which suggests that the antigen functions as a bridge. In many immunizations with a hapten conjugated to a carrier, it has been demonstrated that T cells specific for carrier determinants cooperate with B cells specific for hapten determinants. The effector T cells that cooperate with B cells in antibody formation are those of the

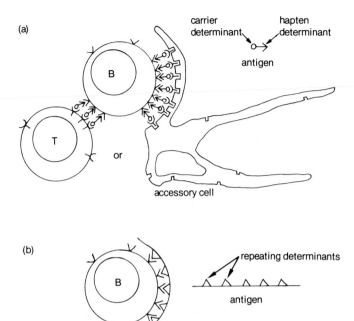

Figure 4–12   Models for T-cell-dependent and T-cell-independent antibody responses (see text). (a) Accessory cells and T cells may be required to present monovalent antigens as a multivalent array to B-cell receptors. (b) Multivalent antigens can activate B cells independently of accessory cells and T cells.

class called T helper (T_H) cells. T_H cells are essential for IgG, IgA, and IgE immune responses; most IgM responses are T_H-cell-independent.

B.   T and B cells require other accessory cells for effective antigen-specific collaboration. Specific T_H cells recognize and respond to antigen only when it is presented by macrophages. Antigen-activated T_H cells also require accessory cells, perhaps macrophages or dendritic reticular cells, to trigger specific B cells (Figure 4–12a). Accessory cells are not antigen-specific, in that they will perform their accessory functions even if derived from a host that cannot respond to the specific antigen. In contrast, antigen-specific T_H and B cells both must be present to produce an antibody response.

C.   Whereas most humoral immune responses are T-cell dependent, antigens that have repeating, identical antigenic determinants (for example, polysaccharides or proteins with identical subunits) can elicit an antibody response in the absence of T cells (Figure 4–12b). If accessory cells or T cells act to convert a monovalent determinant to a multivalent cell-surface array, as suggested in Figure 4–12a, then it would be understandable that a multivalent polymeric antigen could bypass T-cell participation. These T cell-independent antigens stimulate primarily IgM synthesis.

D.   In addition to T_H cells, which stimulate antibody production, there is a class of *suppressor T cells* (T_S cells) that specifically inhibit antibody production. T_S cells are generated by antigenic stimulation, and are antigen-specific in their suppression. It is not yet known whether they act upon antigen-charged accessory cells, T_H cells, or B cells. If they act on lymphocytes, they could recognize either cell-bound antigen or the V-domain (idiotypic) determinants of T- or B-cell receptors.

4–5   Two categories of genes control the B-cell immune response to antigens

The two categories of genes that control the B-cell immune response are *structural genes* for the antibody polypeptide chains and *immune response* (Ir) *genes.*

1.   Structural genes for immunoglobulins belong to three unlinked families (the H chain family, the kappa family, and the lambda chain family). Their properties were discussed in Chapter 2.

2.   Immune response genes have been investigated in various inbred strains of mice. One well-studied locus, the Ir-1 locus, is situated in the middle of the major histocompatibility complex (MHC) and is unlinked to any of the loci that code for antibody polypeptides (Figure 4–13). The Ir-1 locus regulates the amount of IgG (and perhaps IgA and IgE) antibody that is synthesized in response to certain specific antigens that are T-cell dependent. Ir-1 alleles are inherited as dominant or codominant characters. Mice with different Ir-1 alleles can be grouped into two classes: *high responder* mice synthesize 10 to 20 times as much specific IgG antibody as do *low responder* mice. Mice that are high responders to some antigens may be low responders to others. Therefore, Ir genes do not code for general immune responsivity, but show some degree of antigenic specificity.

4–6   Three classes of T cells participate in a cellular immune response

A.   In addition to the helper (T_H) and suppressor (T_S) T-cell functions in a humoral immune response, there are two other T-cell effector functions involved in the generation of cellular immunity. These functions are development of local chronic inflammatory responses by T_D cells and direct lysis of foreign antigenic cells by T_C cells.

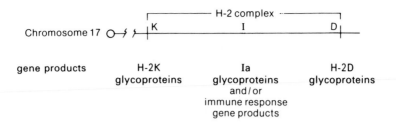

Figure 4–13   A genetic map of the major histocompatibility complex on Chromosome 17 of the mouse. Chromosome 17 carries genes for a variety of different cell-surface molecules, including Ia and the K and D transplantation antigens.

Table 4–2
Classes of effector T cells

Category	Class of cells	Function	Ly phenotype in mice
T_H	T_H	Stimulation of B-cell differentiation	Ly-1
	T_A	Stimulation of T_C precursor cell differentiation	Ly-1
	T_D	Transfer of delayed hypersensitivity	Ly-1
$T_{C,S}$	T_C	Lysis of specific antigenic target cells	Ly-2,3
	T_S	Suppression of immune responses	Ly-2,3

An additional class of T cells, called T_A cells, serves an amplifier function in the maturation of antigen-specific killer T_C cells. T_A cells apparently recognize a macrophage-processed or native cell-surface antigen, and then somehow stimulate T_C-cell precursors that recognize other antigens on the same target cell to proliferate and differentiate to T_C effector cells (Table 4–2).

B.   Serological studies in mice seem to show that the various classes of T cells divide into two major cell categories, which have been designated the T_H category and the $T_{C,S}$ category, distinguishable by their Ly antigens. Table 4–2 lists the various T-cell classes with their functions and serological markers. The classes within the two categories are distinguishable so far only on the basis of their functions. All classes probably include memory cells in addition to effector T cells.

1.   The T_H category, which consists of Ly-1 cells, gives rise to the helper T_H cells, which cooperate with B cells in the humoral response, and to the T_A cells, which play an analogous helper role in killer T_C-cell maturation. The T_H category includes T_D

Table 4–3
Characteristics of some T-cell lymphokines

Lymphokine	Properties
Macrophage chemotactic factor (CF)	Attracts macrophages *in vitro*
Macrophage migration inhibition factor (MIF)	Inhibits macrophage movement *in vitro*
Macrophage aggregation factor (MAF)	Agglutinates macrophages *in vitro*
Lymphocyte blastogenic factor (BF)	Induces lymphocyte DNA synthesis *in vitro*
Lymphotoxin (LT)	Acts *in vitro* as a slow general cytotoxin that spares lymphocytes
Interferon	Prevents viral replication in target cells
Transfer factor	Transfers delayed hypersensitivity to specific antigens from one person to another; dialyzable factor

cells, which are responsible for the establishment of local chronic inflammatory responses such as delayed hypersensitivity.

2. The $T_{C,S}$ category includes suppressor T_S cells as well as precursors of T_C cells. The cells in this category appear to be predominantly of the Ly-2,3 phenotype, although recent experiments have detected both T_C and T_S cells of Ly-1,2,3 phenotype as well.

C. The T cells that mediate delayed hypersensitivity release a variety of polypeptides called *lymphokines* (Table 4–3). Most work on lymphokines so far has been done with animal species in which markers to distinguish T_H and $T_{C,S}$ categories have not been identified. Therefore, production of the various lymphokines cannot yet be assigned to a particular T-cell line.

Lymphokines are believed to attract macrophages and other cells to the site of T-cell interaction with antigen, activate these macrophages to a phagocytic stage of differentiation, and prevent their departure from the site. In addition, other lymphokines are thought to stimulate division of itinerant lymphocytes, recruiting these cells into the chronic inflammatory reaction. The lymphokines also may include agents that nonspecifically damage all cells except lymphocytes, and agents such as *interferon* that prevent intracellular viral multiplication. It is not yet known which of these agents are active *in vivo*, but it has been demonstrated that lymphokines induced in tissue culture will initiate delayed hypersensitivity if injected into the skin, and that antibodies to lymphokines will prevent the expression of delayed hypersensitivity when injected together with antigen.

4-7 Some T cells recognize a gene product of the major histocompatibility complex as well as a specific antigenic determinant

A. In the humoral response to a hapten-carrier antigen, T_H cells recognize and respond to processed carrier antigen on macrophages. These macrophages also express self MHC gene products from the D, K, and I regions as cell-surface glycoproteins, called H-2D, H-2K, and Ia, respectively. T_H-cell receptors recognize both the foreign carrier antigen and Ia glycoproteins on the surface of the presenting macrophage through some type of dual recognition. This recognition of self Ia glycoproteins is required for T_H-macrophage cooperation. By contrast, recognition of macrophage H-2D and H-2K glycoproteins is not required for T_H-macrophage cooperation.

B. In the cellular response to host cells that carry foreign cell-surface antigens (for example, virus-infected cells that carry viral determinants on the cell surface), antigen-specific effector T_C cells recognize, react with, and destroy the antigen-bearing cells. This reaction requires that the effector T_C cells recognize viral antigens in association with self H-2D or H-2K glycoproteins on the target cells. By contrast, recognition of self Ia glycoproteins is not required for T_C-cell–target-cell interaction.

C. These observations suggest that both T_H-macrophage and T_C-target cell interactions involve specific MHC gene products, as well as antigens and antigen-specific receptors. This phenomenon has been termed *associated or dual recognition.* When the immune system is stimulated by exogenous antigen, T_H cells can respond only in the appropriate *context* of I-region gene products and T_C cells can respond only in the appropriate *context* of D/K-region gene products. Neither the mechanism nor the biological function of associated recognition is yet understood, but both raise questions of major importance in understanding the immune system.

4-8 The magnitude and duration of any specific immune response are limited by several mechanisms

Antigenic stimulation causes several categories of cells to proliferate and differentiate, resulting in the generation of several specific and nonspecific effector mechanisms. Uncontrolled continuation of an immune response could lead to pathological lymphoid proliferation, excessive antibody production, and even anti-self reactions. Five major mechanisms are known to control the magnitude and duration of immune responses. The five mechanisms are listed on the next page; misregulation and its pathological consequences will be considered further in Chapters 7 and 8.

1. Effector cells have a lifespan of only a few days, and new effector cells appear only via antigenic stimulation.

2. Antigen is removed as a result of effector-cell functions.

3. Antigen bound to macrophages and reticular cells may become coated with antibodies of high avidity, so that the antigen no longer can stimulate lymphocytes. This process creates a negative-feedback loop that prevents production of a large number of like antibody molecules.

4. Antigenic stimulation of specific T-cell clones may induce specific suppressor T cells, which somehow function to inhibit antigen triggering of other lymphocytes.

5. The V-domains of the antibodies produced in an immune response are themselves potential immunogens to which the organism is not tolerant. If their concentration reaches immunogenic levels, the organism may mount an anti-idiotypic immune response, which may inhibit the lymphocytes that express these V-domains. Thus idiotype-specific T_S and T_C cells and anti-antibodies may be important elements in controlling the magnitude of an immune response.

4-9   Normally the immune system does not respond to self-antigens

A. The immune system can respond in two ways when exposed to an antigen. A positive response leads to differentiation of T and B effector cells, to antibody synthesis, and to immunologic memory. A negative response leads to active suppression or inactivation of specific lymphocytes, and to *tolerance*. Tolerance can be defined as the failure of an organism to mount an immune response against a specific antigen. Normally an organism is tolerant of its own antigens. Immunologic defenses are based on the ability of an organism to distinguish between self and foreign molecules; the effector mechanisms of the immune system, if activated, could destroy self-molecules and cells as effectively as their foreign counterparts. When tolerance to self-antigens is lost, autoimmune disease may ensue.

Both the immune response and tolerance are specific for individual antigens; both are acquired through appropriate antigenic exposure; and both are mediated by lymphocytes. Immunologic memory and tolerance both are active responses of the vertebrate immune system.

B. A vertebrate has the genetic information necessary to synthesize antibodies against self-antigens, but it prevents the expression of this information in effector cells. The mechanism of the tolerance reaction is unclear, but as a consequence of this response, lymphocytes that carry cell-surface receptors specific for self-determinants either are

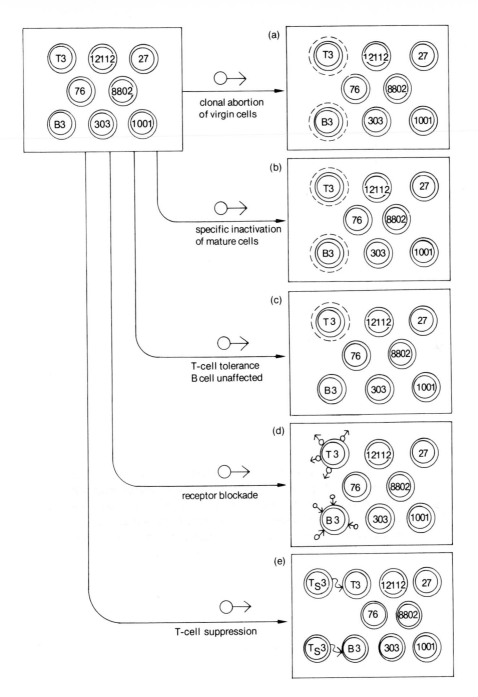

Figure 4–14 Five models for induction of tolerance. The antigen diagramed in the figure has two antigenic determinants, one recognized by B-cell clone 3 and the other by T-cell clone 3. Inactivation of a clone is indicated by a dashed circle. (a) Clonal abortion of virgin lymphocytes, usually accomplished with very low antigen concentrations. (b) Paralysis or inactivation of mature lymphocytes, usually requiring high concentrations of antigen. (c) Tolerance at the level of T cells, but not at the level of B cells. This type of tolerance also prevents B-cell activation for responses that are T-cell dependent. (d) Blockade of receptors by antigen, which leads to paralysis. (e) Activation of specific T$_S$ cells, which prevent specific T$_H$- or B-cell activation.

eliminated or rendered incapable of activation (*paralyzed*) by exposure to these determinants. At an early stage in their differentiation from precursor lymphocytes, B and T cells appear to be particularly sensitive to antigen. Contact at this stage with even low concentrations of self-antigens paralyzes or eliminates immature B and T cells that are self-specific. Since lymphocytes continue to differentiate in the bone marrow and thymus throughout the lifetime of an individual, this process, termed *clonal abortion,* must be an active and continuous check against production of anti-self immunity (Figure 4–14). Maintenance of tolerance requires continued presence of the tolerance-inducing antigen.

C.   During early fetal development the immune system normally is exposed almost exclusively to self-antigens, which react with and paralyze or eliminate all self-specific clones of immature lymphocytes. Later in life it is less clear how the organism distinguishes self from foreign determinants. Some insight into this question has come from experiments on induction of tolerance in mature animals. Certain antigens administered under certain conditions can induce tolerance by eliminating or paralyzing mature lymphocytes (Figure 4–14b).

1.   Mature lymphocytes are far more difficult to inactivate with a tolerance-inducing antigen than are immature lymphocytes. T and B cells of adult animals respond differently to the induction of tolerance. Very low (subimmunogenic) doses of an appropriate antigen can inactivate only T cells (*low zone tolerance*), whereas high doses produce a more rapid and prolonged tolerance in T cells than in B cells. Since B and T cells must cooperate to produce most humoral immune responses, tolerance in either cell type can block the synthesis of specific antibodies (Figure 4–14c).

2.   The form of an antigen may determine whether it elicits a positive or a negative immune response. Aggregated protein antigens, for example, are always immunogenic at all concentrations, whereas soluble monomeric forms of the same determinants may be immunogenic or tolerance-inducing (*tolerogenic*). In general, a high dose of a monomeric antigen favors a negative response. Some self-antigens always will be present at higher levels than most foreign antigens. Conceivably, the immune system also has mechanisms for presenting self-antigens in more tolerogenic forms.

3.   One type of experimentally induced tolerance is somewhat better understood and may have important clinical applications. Very high doses of polysaccharide antigens cause paralysis of most of the antigen-specific B cells by binding to all their surface receptors (Figure 4–14d). This binding is reversible, but if the antigen is present at high enough levels it nevertheless can prevent B-cell activation by a mechanism that is still unknown. A small

amount of humoral antibody is produced, but then is absorbed by the excess of antigen.

Unnatural D-isomers of polypeptide antigens also induce tolerance by blockade of B-cell receptors. This blockade is irreversible, because mammals lack proteases that can degrade polypeptides of D-amino acids. This situation can be exploited clinically to induce tolerance to an allergen or a drug to which a patient normally mounts an immune response. Penicillin, for example, can be linked chemically to a D-polypeptide. When the resulting compound is injected in high doses into a sensitive individual, the penicillin-specific B-cell receptors become blockaded, and the allergic reaction to penicillin is eliminated.

4. Induction of tolerance in later life may be a cooperative phenomenon, rather than a direct antigen-mediated elimination or paralysis of reactive clones. Selective activation of T_S cells suppresses immune responses to specific antigens; this process is operationally equivalent to tolerance (Figure 4–14e). The two types of tolerance may be distinguished by mixing lymphocytes from a tolerant host with lymphocytes from a normal host. Tolerance mediated by T_S cells will prevent normal lymphocytes from reacting to the tolerance-inducing antigen, whereas clonal deletion or clonal abortion leaves a tolerant cell population that will not transfer tolerance to normal lymphocytes. Both types of tolerance have been demonstrated by this test.

Selected Bibliography

Burnet, F. M. (Ed.), *Immunology,* W. H. Freeman and Company, San Francisco, 1976. Clearly illustrated, well-written Scientific American articles with incisive and imaginative mini-articles by the editor.

Katz, D. H., *Lymphocyte Differentiation, Recognition, and Regulation,* Academic Press, New York, 1977. A comprehensive and up-to-date description of the cells and cellular interactions involved in the immune response.

Mayer, M., "The complement system," *Sci. Am.* **229,** 54 (1973).

McDevitt, H. O., "The evolution of the genes in the major histocompatibility complex," *Fed. Proceedings* **35,** 2168 (1976). This paper presents the discovery of MHC-linked immune response genes and the current understanding of entities recognized by T-cell receptors.

Spiegelberg, H. L., "Biological activities of immunoglobulins of different classes and subclasses," *Adv. Immunol.* **259,** 19 (1974). This article describes recent knowledge of several of the effector mechanisms triggered by combination of antibodies with target antigens.

Exercises

4–1   Indicate whether each of the following statements is true or false. Explain the error in each statement you consider to be false.

F   (a)   In a secondary immune response, IgM is the major class of antibody synthesized.

F   (b)   Antibodies generally do not react with self molecules because genes that code for self-antibodies are not inherited.

F   (c)   Antigenic stimulation of macrophages in the thymus will trigger their differentiation into T cells.

F   (d)   Activation of the third component of complement, C3, occurs only when an antigen interacts with specific antibody of a class that can fix complement.

T   (e)   Delayed hypersensitivity lesions contain cellular infiltrates composed of lymphocytes and macrophages.

F   (f)   In the presence of antigen, a purified population of T and B cells may cooperate *in vitro* to produce a B-cell immune response.

F   (g)   Genes that code for antibody combining-site specificities, and thereby control the immune response to specific antigens, are linked to MHC genes.

T   (h)   Killer cells may derive from either T-cell or macrophage lineages.

4–2   Supply the missing word or words in each of the following statements.

(a)   The major class of antibody synthesized in a _secondary_ immune response is IgG.

(b)   _Blast transformation_ is the process whereby a lymphocyte undergoes an antigen-driven differentiation.

(c)   The B-cell response usually requires the cooperation of _T_H cells_, _B cell_, and _macrophages_.

(d)   T-cell-independent antigens evoke the synthesis of antibody of the _IgM_ class.

(e)   Genes that regulate the antibody response to many antigens and are linked to the major histocompatibility genes of the mouse are called _Immune response_ genes.

(f)   Administration of Dnp-D (glu,lys) to mice will lead to Dnp tolerance caused by B lymphocyte _receptor blockade_.

(g)   Mast cells possess surface receptors for _IgE_ antibodies.

(h)   _IgG_ immunoglobulins are transported across the placental barrier to the fetus.

Answers are given on pages 155–156.

5 IMMUNOASSAY AND IMMUNODIAGNOSIS

Assays for the measurement of antibody–antigen reactions have been instrumental in the development of the science of immunology. Moreover, immunoassays have revolutionized modern medicine by allowing rapid and precise detection of even minute quantities of clinically significant molecules in human tissues or serum. This chapter considers the basic principles that underlie immunoassay techniques.

Essential Concepts

5-1 Antigen–antibody reactions can be measured by the formation of insoluble complexes

A.   Precipitation of antigen–antibody complexes from solution (the *precipitin* reaction) can be used to estimate the amount of antigen or antibody in a test sample. Multivalent antigens may interact with multivalent antibodies to form large insoluble lattices (Figure 5–1a) or small soluble complexes (Figure 5–1b,c). When large antigen–antibody complexes precipitate out of solution, the amount of antigen and antibody precipitated can be measured.

1.   Complexes precipitate most completely at roughly equal concentrations of antigen and antibody. Excess antibody allows single antigen molecules to be coated by several antibodies, and thus prevents lattice formation (Figure 5–1b). Excess antigen causes saturation of all antibody-combining sites with different antigen molecules, again preventing lattice formation (Figure 5–1c). In the precipitin assay, a fixed quantity of antiserum is reacted with increasing concentrations of antigen, and the amounts of antibody or antigen in the precipitate are measured either

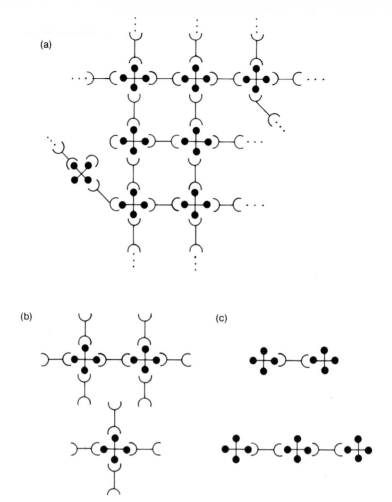

Figure 5–1 Complexes of antibody with antigen. Antigenic determinants are represented as solid circles and the antibody-binding sites that recognize them as open semicircles. (a) Lattice formulation near the equivalence point. (b) Soluble complexes in the presence of excess antibody. (c) Soluble complexes in the presence of excess antigen. [Adapted from I. Roitt, *Essential Immunology,* 2nd ed., Blackwell, London, 1974, p. 6]

chemically, by various assays for protein or carbohydrate; radiochemically, if either reactant is labeled with a radioisotope; or biologically, if the antigen exhibits, for example, a toxic or enzymatic activity that can be measured in the soluble fraction before and after precipitation.

2. Figure 5–2 shows a typical *precipitin curve* that might be obtained with standard solutions of antigen and antibody. In the example shown, 0.1-ml samples of antihemoglobin antiserum are added to increasing amounts of pure hemoglobin in a series of tubes (Figure 5–2a). These mixtures are incubated, and the

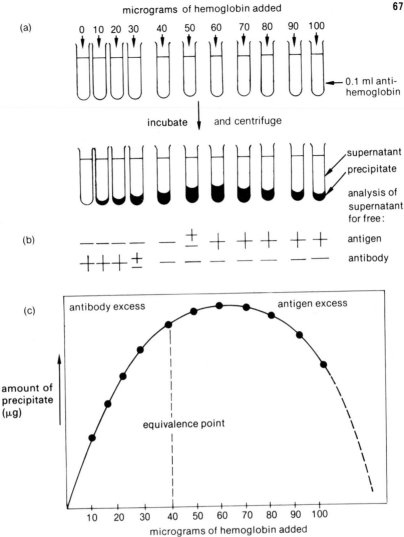

Figure 5–2 A precipitin curve for the reaction of hemoglobin with anti-hemoglobin. (a) Mixing of 0.1-ml aliquots of anti-hemoglobin with increasing amounts of hemoglobin. (b) Separation of immune precipitate and supernatant fraction by centrifugation. (c) Precipitin curve plot as amount of precipitate versus amount of antigen added. See text for details. [Adapted from I. Roitt, *Essential Immunology*, 2nd ed., Blackwell, London, 1974, p. 5.]

resulting precipitates are collected by centrifugation and assayed. The supernatant fractions are assayed for presence of residual antibody and antigen (Figure 5–2b). The amounts of the precipitates then are plotted against the amounts of antigens added (Figure 5–2c). The tube in which neither antigen nor antibody is found in the supernatant fraction defines the *equivalence point* of the precipitin curve. This point generally does not correspond to the point of maximum precipitation, which usually occurs at a slight weight excess of antigen.

Once such a standard curve is prepared, precipitin assays can be used to estimate amounts of the antigen in test samples of unknown concentration. Using the standard antiserum in this example, equivalence will be reached when the test sample added contains 40 μg of hemoglobin. Similar assays may be used to compare other serum samples to the standard antiserum; if dilutions of a test serum are added to tubes that each contain 40 μg of hemoglobin, the equivalence point will define the dilution of test serum in which the antibody concentration is the same as in the standard serum.

B.   Antigen–antibody precipitates also can be conveniently formed and observed by allowing one reactant to diffuse into a gelatinous medium, such as agar, that contains the other. In the widely used *Ouchterlony double-diffusion* technique, antigen and antibody samples are placed in small wells cut into an agar slab. The molecules of each diffuse out of their respective wells into the agar at a rate inversely proportional to their molecular weights, if the molecules have no affinity for the agar itself. If an antigen reacts with an antibody, then a line of precipitation (*precipitin* line) will form where the two reactants diffuse together.

1.   A diagram of such a test is shown in Figure 5–3. The antibody is a rabbit antibody against the κ light chain of mouse immunoglobulin. The κ light chain is a common element of the three

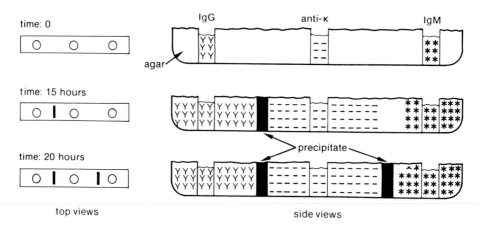

Figure 5–3   Ouchterlony double diffusion in an agar slab. The center well contains antibody against mouse κ chains. The outer wells contain IgM and IgG as antigens, both of which have κ chains which will complex with the antibody (see text for details).

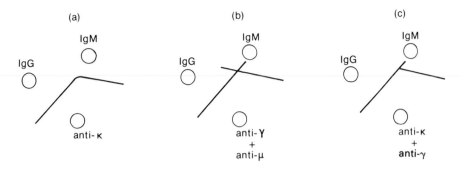

Figure 5–4   An Ouchterlony double diffusion analysis of related antigens. (a) Reaction of identity. (b) Reaction of nonidentity. (c) Reaction of partial identity (see text for details).

immunoglobulin classes IgG, IgA, and IgM. IgG and IgM, with molecular weights of 160,000 and 900,000, respectively, are used as test antigens in the experiment. The IgG and the anti-κ antibodies diffuse toward one another at equal rates and form a precipitate near the point at which the antibody and IgG fronts meet. The anti-κ front continues to diffuse and a second precipitate forms when the anti-κ antibody meets the more slowly diffusing IgM.

2.   If serial dilutions of an antigen, for example IgG, are tested against anti-κ antibody in this system, the distance between the antigen well and the precipitin line will vary with antigen concentration. Because the diffusion gradient of anti-κ is constant, the location of the precipitin line will be determined by the diffusion gradient of the antigen, which will depend upon its concentration in the well. Accordingly, this assay can be used to compare antigen concentrations in different samples.

3.   The Ouchterlony technique can be used to determine whether two antigens are different or identical, or whether they share some but not all antigenic determinants. Three such experiments are shown in Figure 5–4.

In Experiment (a), anti-κ antibody forms a single continuous precipitin line equidistant from both antigen wells, thereby showing that the two antigen samples cannot be distinguished by this antiserum. This result is called a *reaction of identity*.

In Experiment (b), the antibody well contains a mixture of antibodies against IgG heavy chains (anti-γ) and IgM heavy chains (anti-μ). Because anti-μ precipitates IgM but not IgG, the antibodies migrate through the IgG precipitin line and precipitate IgM on the other side. The reverse is true for the anti-γ antibodies, which precipitate IgG but not IgM. The resulting pattern of crossed

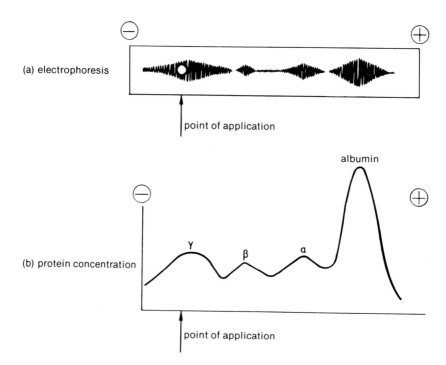

(a) electrophoresis

point of application

(b) protein concentration

albumin

γ

β

α

point of application

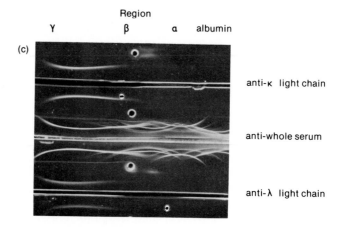

Region

γ   β   α   albumin

(c)

anti-κ light chain

anti-whole serum

anti-λ light chain

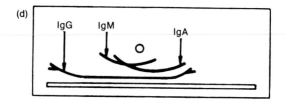

(d)

IgG   IgM   IgA

precipitin lines indicates that the antibody recognizes different determinants on the two antigens. This result is termed a *reaction of nonidentity*.

In Experiment (c), the antibody well contains a mixture of anti-κ and anti-γ antibodies. The anti-κ precipitates both IgG and IgM, forming a continuous precipitin line. The anti-γ, however, migrates through the IgM zone to precipitate IgG behind it, thereby forming a spur. This result indicates that the antibody recognizes determinants in the left antigen well that are not present in the right well. This result is termed a *reaction of partial identity*.

C. The related technique of *immunoelectrophoresis* provides improved resolution for complex samples by combining electrophoresis of antigens in one dimension with subsequent double diffusion of antibodies and separated antigens in a second dimension. The experimental system is diagramed in Figure 5–5. In this example the mixture of antigens to be analyzed is a whole serum.

1. Separation of serum components by gel electrophoresis alone is shown in Figure 5–5a. A serum sample is placed in the well near one end of a suitably buffered gel slab, and an electrical current is applied across the gel. The various serum components migrate through the gel at rates proportional to their charge / mass ratios. Four major classes of proteins are resolved as distinct components: albumins migrate most rapidly, followed by α-, β-, and γ-globulins. The amount of protein at each point in the gel can be determined by staining and measurement of light absorption (Figure 5–5b). All immunoglobulins are found in the γ- or β-globulin fractions.

2. An immunoelectrophoresis experiment is illustrated in Figure 5–5c. Four samples of serum are placed in wells near the left side of a large gel slab and are subjected to electrophoresis in parallel. Slots then are cut into the gel parallel to the direction

⟵ **Figure 5–5** Immunoelectrophoresis in an agar slab. (a) A protein sample is placed in a hole in an agarose gel, which is then subjected to an electric field. The relative migration of various proteins is illustrated. (b) A quantitative assessment of the amount of protein that migrates across the gel. Four categories of proteins are noted: albumin, α-globulins, β-globulins, and γ-globulins. Most antibodies are γ-globulins. (c) Following electrophoresis, antibodies to serum protein are placed in the horizontal slot, and the antibodies and separated serum protein antigens diffuse toward each other to form precipitin lines. Anti-whole serum, placed in the center slot, forms a large number of precipitin lines with various serum components. Anti-κ serum, placed in the top slot, reveals only γ-globulins that contain κ light chains. Notice that only a single line is formed, demonstrating complete absorption of anti-κ by the first immunoglobulin it meets. Anti-λ serum, placed in the bottom slot, detects γ-globulins that contain λ chains. (d) An idealized anti-whole serum pattern, showing the relative positions of IgG, IgM, and IgA.

of electrophoresis and filled with various test antibody preparations. The antibodies and the separated antigenic components diffuse toward each other through the gel and form precipitin lines that indicate which of the antigenic serum components are reactive with the various antibodies. An idealized drawing of the precipitin lines that would be obtained with IgM, IgG, and IgA as antigens with anti-whole serum antibody is shown in Figure 5–5d.

D.   Antigen-antibody complex formation can be measured by quantitatively precipitating immunoglobulins under conditions that will not precipitate free antigen, and then determining the amount of bound antigen in the precipitate.

1. The *Farr assay* employs 50% ammonium sulfate, which precipitates most immunoglobulins but not haptens and many proteins. Figure 5–6a shows the results of a typical Farr assay with antiserum against the hapten *digoxin,* a drug that commonly is used to regulate the heart action of cardiac disease patients. For convenience the hapten is labeled radioactively. Tests with a constant amount of the hapten in increasing dilutions of antiserum define the antibody concentration sufficient to precipitate 50% of the hapten under these conditions. Once such a standard curve is available, it can be used to compare the anti-digoxin antibody titer of other serum samples relative to that of the standard.

Precipitation also can be carried out with an immunoglobulin-specific antibody from another species (*heterologous anti-immunoglobulin*). For example, if the specific antibody used for antigen–antibody complex formation is from a rabbit, it can be precipitated by a goat antibody specific for rabbit immunoglobulin, added at a concentration that gives maximum precipitation.

2. The preceding techniques also can be used to measure competitive binding for *quantitative radioimmunoassay* of a known antigen in the presence of many other components. An example is the clinically important method used to monitor serum levels of digoxin. Monitoring is crucial because the drug is highly toxic at levels not far above the therapeutic serum concentration. For the assay, radiolabeled digoxin is incubated with sufficient digoxin-specific antibody to precipitate 70–90% of the radioactivity in the Farr assay. A standard curve then is prepared by adding known amounts of unlabeled digoxin to the incubation mixture and measuring the decrease of radioactivity in the precipitate due to competition between labeled and unlabeled antigen for the antibody-binding sites (Figure 5–6b). Samples of serum from patients receiving digoxin then can be added to

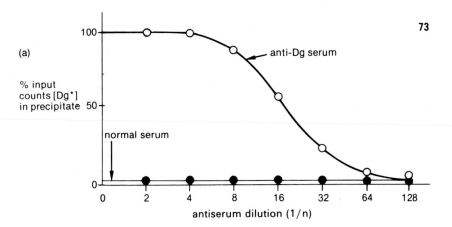

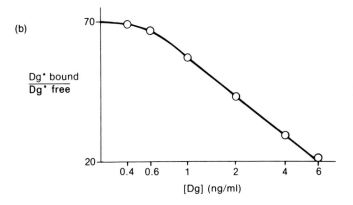

Figure 5–6 (a) Measurement of antibody–hapten complex formation using the Farr assay. A standard amount of labeled digoxin (Dg*) is added to each of a series of two-fold dilutions of anti-digoxin antiserum. After several hours, free antibody and antibody–hapten complex are precipitated by bringing the solution to 50% saturation with ammonium sulfate. The percentage of radioactivity in the precipitate then is plotted against serum dilution. (b) A competitive radioimmunoassay using the Farr technique. The serum dilution that gives approximately 70% precipitation in (a) is added to a series of tubes that contain the standard amount of labeled digoxin and varying concentrations (0.4 to 6 ng/ml) of unlabeled digoxin. A standard curve is prepared by plotting the ratio of bound to free labeled digoxin against nanograms of unlabeled dixogin added. This standard curve then can be used to determine the concentration of unlabeled digoxin in samples of patient's serum. Current radioimmunoassays for digoxin take advantage of the fact that dextran-coated charcoal particles will bind free but not antibody-bound digoxin.

the assay mixture, and their digoxin content can be estimated from the observed decrease in bound radioactivity, using the standard curve.

3. Immunoprecipitation can be used not only analytically, but also as a highly specific preparative technique. Antibody specific for one component in a complex mixture can be used to precipitate the component either directly, using ammonium sulfate, or indirectly, using an appropriate heterologous anti-immunoglobulin. The purified component then can be eluted from the precipitate, often by treatment with a competing hapten, a protein denaturant, or a buffer of low pH.

5-2   The strength of interaction between antigens and antibodies can be measured

A.   The affinity of antibody-binding sites for cognate monovalent antigens can vary widely. Binding can be described by Equation 5-1,

$$\text{Ag} + \text{Ab} \underset{k_2}{\overset{k_1}{\rightleftharpoons}} \text{Ag–Ab} \tag{5-1}$$

in which Ag, Ab, and Ag–Ab represent unbound antigenic determinants, antibody-binding sites, and bound antigenic determinants, respectively, and k_1 and k_2 are rate constants for the association and dissociation reactions, respectively. The antigen–antibody *affinity* in such a reaction can be measured as the ratio of complexed to free reactants at equilibrium. The affinity constant, K, is defined by Equation 5-2:

$$K = \frac{[\text{Ag–Ab}]}{[\text{Ag}]\,[\text{Ab}]} \tag{5-2}$$

K also is equal to k_1/k_2. Because K is an *association* constant, its value will be high for high-affinity complexes and low for low-affinity complexes. Typical K values vary from 10^5 to 10^{11} liters per mole.

> **1.**   Like any equilibrium constant, K is related to the standard free energy change of the binding reaction at pH 7 ($\Delta G_0'$) in kilocalories per mole, by Equation 5-3,
>
> $$\Delta G_0' = -\text{RT}\,\ln K \tag{5-3}$$
>
> in which R is the gas constant (0.00198 kilocalorie per mole per degree) and T is the absolute temperature, 298°K.
>
> **2.**   The affinity of an antibody-binding site for a monovalent hapten can be measured by *equilibrium dialysis* (Figure 5-7). A concentrated solution of antibody in a dialysis sac, which is permeable to hapten but not to antibodies, is placed in a known volume of buffer that contains hapten at a concentration in the range of $1/K$. At equilibrium, the concentrations of bound plus free hapten inside the sac [I] and free hapten outside the sac [O] will depend upon the concentration and average affinity of the antibodies inside the sac.

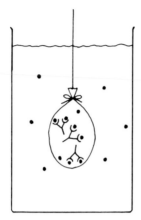

Figure 5–7   Equilibrium dialysis. A concentrated solution of antibodies (—⟨) against a hapten (●) is placed in a sac of dialysis tubing which is permeable to the hapten but not to the antibodies, and the sac is suspended in a known volume of hapten solution. When the system reaches equilibrium, the concentration of free hapten will be the same throughout, but the sac will contain bound hapten as well. The difference in total hapten concentration inside and outside the sac can be measured and used to calculate the average affinity of the antibodies for the hapten (see text).

Using equilibrium dialysis, one can determine both the average association constant, K, and the antibody valence, n, from the relationship described in Equation 5–4,

$$\frac{r}{c} = Kn - Kr \tag{5-4}$$

in which r is the ratio of moles of hapten bound per mole of antibody and c is the concentration of unbound hapten $(= [O])$. The moles of hapten bound are determined by subtracting $[O]$ from $[I]$. Since Kn is a constant, a plot of r/c versus r for different hapten concentrations will approximate a straight line with slope $-K$, so that the association constant K can be determined as the negative of the slope, and the antibody valence as the r intercept at infinite hapten concentration.

B.   Binding of antibody to a typical multivalent antigen is not as easily defined as binding to a monovalent hapten. Because several different affinities may be involved, the term *avidity* is used to designate the strength of multivalent antigen binding. The kinetics of such binding are complex, because binding of one antigenic determinant affects the rates of binding of others on the same molecule. The net avidity of an antibody–multivalent antigen interaction is a complex function of the valences of both reactants and the affinities of the various determinants involved.

5-3   Binding of antibodies to cell-surface antigens can be detected in several ways

A.   Cells can be agglutinated by cross-linking with antibodies. Cell agglutination is the basis for several widely used assays.

    1.   An agglutination assay is used commonly for the typing of human blood. Human red blood cells may carry the cell-surface antigens A and B, which define the well-known blood groups, AB, A, B, and O. The human blood-group substances called the ABO antigens are cell-surface oligosaccharides whose genetics and chemistry are better understood than those of any other cell-surface carbohydrate system. These blood-group oligosaccharides are attached to glycolipids in the plasma membranes of red blood cells and other human cells. In addition, they may be attached to soluble glycoproteins that are found in secretions such as saliva, tears, and gastric juice. All humans express the blood-group antigens on cell membranes whereas only individuals who carry a secretor gene (Se) express these antigens as glycoproteins in their secretions.

    Blood-group specificities related to the ABO system can be detected by ''natural'' antibodies present in humans who lack the corresponding cell-surface antigens. All natural antibodies to these blood-group antigens are IgM immunoglobulins. The relationships among ABO phenotypes, genotypes, and natural serum antibodies are given in Table 5-1. If antibody specific for blood group A antigens is reacted with red cells that carry group A antigens, the resulting agglutination visibly alters the normal settling pattern of the cells in a test tube or a well of a test tray (Figure 5-8). If the cells do not carry group A antigens,

Table 5-1

Relation between genotype, red blood cell antigens, and serum antibodies in the ABO blood-group system

Blood group (phenotype)	Genotype	Antigen on red cell	Antibodies in serum
A	AA AO	A	anti-B
B	BB BO	B	anti-A
AB	AB	AB	neither anti-A nor anti-B
O	OO	—	anti-A and anti-B

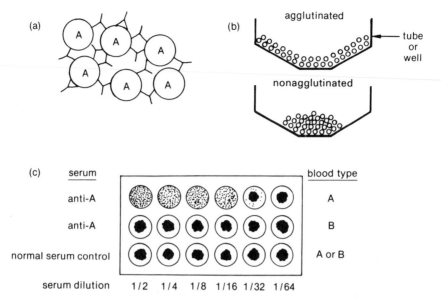

Figure 5–8 The red-cell agglutination assay for typing of human blood groups. (a) At the microscopic level, divalent anti-A antibodies cross-link red cells that carry A antigen to form a lattice of agglutinated cells. (b) Agglutination affects the settling pattern of cells in a test tube or in the well of a test tray. (c) This effect can be exploited to type blood cells for A antigen using a tray test with several dilutions of anti-A serum.

then no agglutination is observed. Type A and type B blood cells are identified as being agglutinated only by specific anti-A and anti-B antibodies, respectively. Type AB cells are agglutinated by both specific antibodies, and type O cells by neither. Thus all four blood types of the ABO system can be identified by these simple tests. Agglutination is also used to type humans for other blood group systems, such as Rh and Lewis. Knowledge of blood types allows transfusions to be made only with serologically compatible blood, thereby avoiding induction of agglutinating antibodies in the recipient.

2. The cell-agglutination technique can be used to assay antibodies specific for antigens that either are normally present on a cell surface or can be coupled artificially to a cell surface. Coupling can be accomplished by treating red cells to promote electrostatic binding of proteins to their surfaces, or by chemically cross-linking antigens to red cells. Appropriate dilutions of the unknown antibody sample are incubated with the antigen-bearing test cells, and the antibody concentration (*titer*) is determined by comparing the resulting agglutination responses to those obtained with a standard antibody sample of known titer.

3. The sensitivity of the agglutination reaction with antibody can be increased markedly by incubation with a heterologous anti-immunoglobulin. This technique, known as the Coombs test, is particularly useful when agglutination by the first test antibody is inefficient; nonagglutinated cells that have bound the first antibody will be agglutinated by the second (Figure 5–9).

4. Competitive inhibition of cell-agglutination reactions can be used to assay free antigens identical to those on the surface of a target cell. For example, if an agglutination reaction is set up with an amount of antibody just sufficient to agglutinate visibly, then minute amounts of competing free antigen in test samples can be detected by preincubating with the antibody and then testing for inhibition of agglutination (Figure 5–10).

B. Cells that carry antibodies bound to cell-surface antigens may be lysed by complement. The ability of the terminal steps in the complement sequence to lyse target cells is the basis for a number of widely used assays for antigen–antibody reactions. Guinea pig serum is a commonly used source of complement.

1. Complement-mediated lysis of target cells, usually red blood cells, can be measured in a variety of ways. Lysis can be followed directly by decrease in optical density of a cell suspension, or

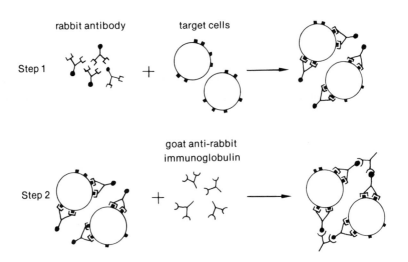

Figure 5–9 Use of a heterologous anti-immunoglobulin to agglutinate cells complexed with a non-agglutinating antibody. Some antibodies that bind to the cell surface are ineffective in promoting agglutination (Step 1). If antibodies directed against the first antibodies then are added to the system, agglutination occurs (Step 2). This technique, called the Coombs test, often is used in clinical laboratories to detect cell-surface antigens and antibody-coated red cells.

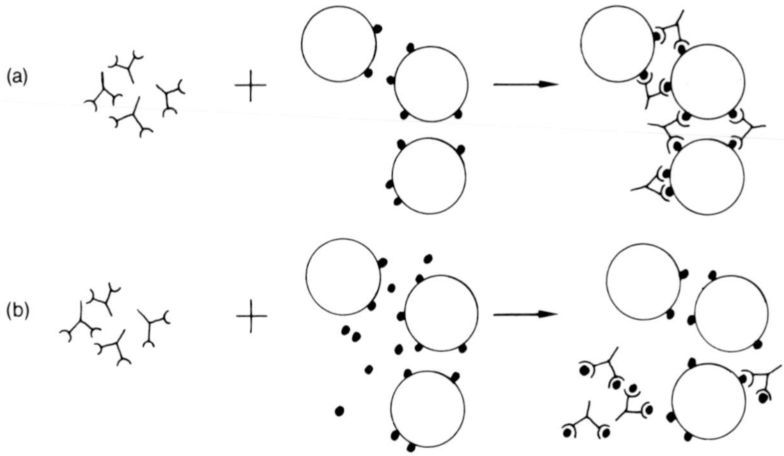

Figure 5–10   Competitive inhibition between cell-bound and free antigens. (a) Cells are agglutinated by antibodies against a cell-bound antigen. (b) Cells are not agglutinated when competing free antigen is present.

by release of cell components that normally are confined internally, such as hemoglobin, enzymes, or a previously introduced isotope such as ^{51}Cr. Alternatively, loss of membrane integrity can be followed by failure to exclude vital dyes such as trypan blue or eosin, or by failure to concentrate compounds such as fluorescein diacetate that are converted to fluorescent derivatives (fluorescein in this example) by intracellular enzymes.

2.   Complement-mediated lysis can be used as an assay for humoral antibodies specific for antigens on the surface of target cells. As in the agglutination assays, these antigens either may be intrinsic membrane components or may be coupled artificially to target cells. In the assay, a sample to be tested for antibody is incubated with antigen-bearing target cells; complement then is added, and cell lysis or membrane disruption is measured (Figure 5–11). If antibody is limiting, the degree of lysis will be a function of the sample's antibody concentration, which can be determined by comparison with a previously prepared standard curve that indicates degree of lysis as a function of known antibody concentration.

The foregoing procedure can detect only antibodies of the complement-activating classes of immunoglobulins: IgM and most IgG subclasses. Nonactivating antibodies can be detected by including an additional step. Following incubation with the test antibody sample, the cells are further incubated with a heterologous anti-immunoglobulin of a complement-activating class prior

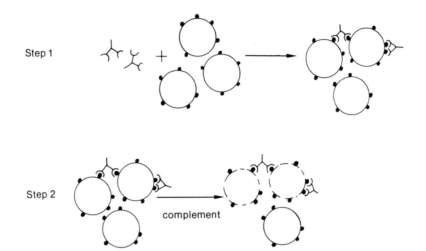

Step 1

Step 2

complement

Figure 5–11 Complement-mediated cell lysis as an assay for antibody binding to cell-surface antigens. Target cells are preincubated with limiting amounts of antibody (Step 1) and then treated with complement (Step 2), which lyses only cells to which antibody has bound.

to addition of complement. Cell-bound test antibodies will in turn bind the heterologous anti-immunoglobulin to produce complexes that will trigger complement-mediated cell lysis.

3. Complement-mediated lysis also can be used as an assay for lymphoid cells that produce antibodies specific to a cell-surface antigen (the *Jerne plaque assay*). An excess of red blood cells bearing the target antigen is mixed with a suspension of the lymphoid cells to be assayed, plated as a monolayer on a suitable surface, and incubated to allow plasma cells to release their immunoglobulins (Figure 5–12a). The monolayer then is overlaid with complement, which creates a zone of red cell lysis (plaque) around any plasma cell that has secreted specific antibody (Figure 5–12b). The number of antibody-producing cells in the suspension thus will be indicated by the number of plaques observed in the monolayer. Cells producing antibodies that do not activate complement also can be assayed, by treating the monolayer of red cells and lymphoid cells with an appropriate heterologous anti-immunoglobulin prior to addition of complement. Specificity of the assay may be validated by demonstrating that preincubation of the lymphoid cell suspension with a free form of the target antigen prevents subsequent plaque formation, and relative estimates of antigen–antibody avidity may be obtained by adding varying amounts of a competing soluble antigen to the test dish.

4. Any complex of a soluble antigen with a complement-activating antibody can be assayed by the technique of *complement*

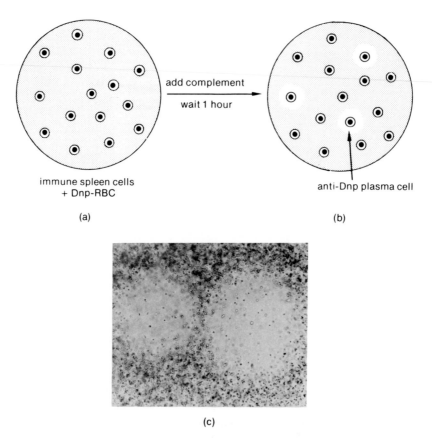

(a)   (b)

(c)

Figure 5–12   The Jerne plaque assay for antibody-producing cells. In the example shown, spleen cells from a mouse that had been immunized with Dnp coupled to a carrier protein were mixed with melted agar and enough red blood cells bearing coupled Dnp groups to give a continuous lawn of cells when poured onto an agar plate. Anti-Dnp-specific plasma cells among the spleen cells continue to produce anti-Dnp antibodies, which bind to surrounding red blood cells (a). When complement is added, these cells lyse to form a plaque, which indicates the presence of an anti-Dnp-specific plasma cell (b). A photomicrograph of two plaques is shown in (c). The assay provides a convenient method for quantitating the antigen-specific plasma cells produced in an immune response.

fixation. This assay is based on the principle that complement that has been activated (fixed) by soluble antigen–antibody complexes will be unavailable for subsequent complement-mediated cell lysis. A limiting amount of complement, known to cause lysis of a certain number of red blood cells treated with anti-red-blood-cell antibody, is incubated with the test antigen and a sample of the antibody preparation to be assayed. The mixture then is added to a suspension of antibody-treated red blood cells, and its capacity to cause lysis is assayed. Given

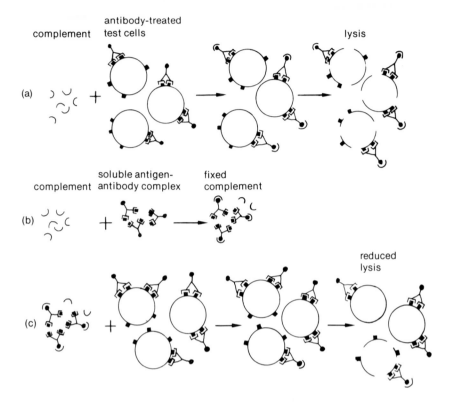

Figure 5–13 Complement fixation by soluble antigen–antibody complexes. (a) Complement lyses antibody-treated test cells. (b) Complement preincubated with soluble antigen–antibody complexes binds to the complexes. (c) Fewer complement molecules are available in the preincubated preparation to lyse antibody-treated test cells.

appropriate controls to show that the test antigen alone does not affect complement activity, reduced red blood cell lysis indicates the presence of antibody specific for test antigen in the sample assayed (Figure 5–13). The titer of this antibody can be determined quantitatively by comparison with an appropriate standard curve prepared using specific antibody of known titer.

5. An important clinical procedure is the assay of complement levels in human serum by determining the ability of serum samples to mediate lysis of red blood cells treated with specific antibodies. A sudden drop in serum complement activity usually indicates complement activation *in vivo*, presumably as the result of antigen–antibody reactions. In patients with some immunological diseases, a fall in complement activity usually heralds an immunologic crisis.

C.   Cellular antigens can be detected directly using specific antibodies with attached fluorescent, radioactive, enzymatic, or electron-opaque markers. This approach is valuable both for determining the locations of antigenic structural components in basic research on cell and tissue ultrastructure, and for identifying characteristic disease-related antigens in clinical diagnosis.

    1. Fluorescent compounds (fluorochromes), such as fluorescein and rhodamine, can be coupled chemically to antibodies without affecting antigen binding. When activated by illumination with light of an appropriate wavelength, the antibody-bound fluorochrome absorbs light energy, attains an excited state, and then returns to its ground state by emitting light at a characteristic longer wavelength. Fluorescein is excited at 490 nm and emits at 517 nm to give a yellow-green fluorescence. Rhodamine is excited at 515 nm and emits at 546 nm to give a red fluorescence. A fluorescence microscope equipped with the appropriate excitatory light source and filters allows visualization of fluorochrome-labeled antibodies bound specifically to cells and tissues (Figure 5–14a). The presence of two different antigens can be monitored simultaneously using two specific antibodies labeled with fluorochromes that fluoresce at different wave-

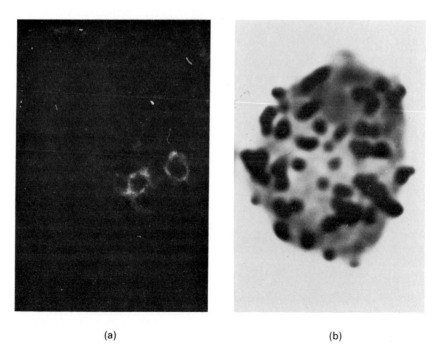

(a)   (b)

Figure 5–14 The direct visualization of antibody—antigen complexes. (a) Immunoflorescence identification of T lymphocytes in a lymph node B-cell region. [Photograph by G. Gutman.] (b) Autoradiography of a lymphocyte with ^{125}I-bound antibody. [Photograph by G. Edelman.]

lengths. This technique often is used in urgent diagnosis of pathogenic organisms from an infected focus.

2. Antibodies also can be labeled radioisotopically without destroying their abilities to bind antigen. A common technique is chemical- or enzyme-catalyzed iodination of tyrosine side chains on the antibody molecule, using either of two radioactive isotopes of iodine, ^{125}I or ^{131}I. Both these isotopes are γ-emitters, whose presence can be detected in a gamma counter. Both isotopes also emit short-range ionizing particles (Auger electrons and β particles, respectively) which can be detected photographically by *radioautography*, taking advantage of the capacity of the emitted ionizing radiation to expose a photographic emulsion locally. If antigen-bearing cells are exposed to a specific labeled antibody and then washed to remove unbound molecules, gamma counting allows precise quantitation of the amount of antibody

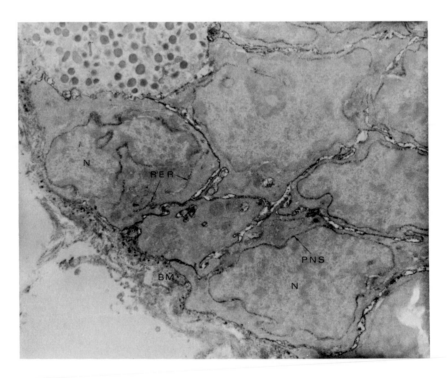

Figure 5–15 Horseradish peroxidase-coupled antibody to human secretory component (SC) reveals the subcellular locations of SC molecules to be the perinuclear space (PNS), the plasma membrane, and the rough endoplasmic reticulum (RER) of human small intestinal epithelial cells (N, nucleus; BM, basement membrane). [From W. R. Brown, Y. Isobe, and P. Nakane.]

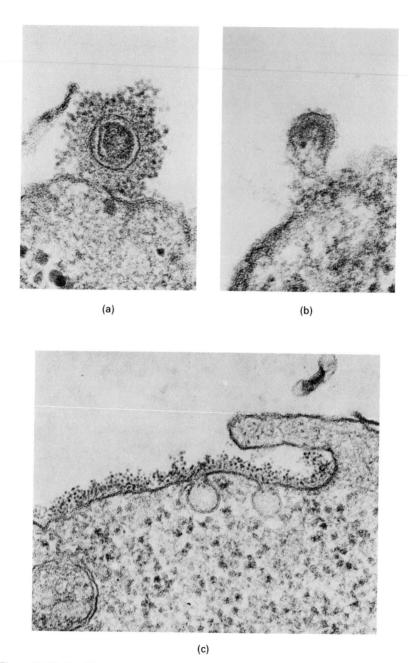

(a)   (b)

(c)

Figure 5–16   Ferritin-coupled antibody to mouse leukemia virus antigens is used to demonstrate that (1) a mouse virus carries these antigens; (b) a cat virus does not; (c) these antigens may be expressed on regions of a cell membrane. [From L. Oshiro, J. A. Levy, J. L. Riggs, and E. H. Lennette, *J. Gen. Virol.* **35,** 317 (1977). ©1977 by Cambridge University Press.]

taken up by the cell population. Radioautography provides additional information. If the treated cells are spread on a suitable surface, covered with a photographic emulsion, and stored in the dark to allow exposure to the emitted ionizing radiation, then silver grains will appear on the developed film as an "autograph" that indicates the locations of bound antibodies. In this manner the distribution and number of antibody molecules bound to individual cells in the population can be determined (Figure 5–14b). The same technique can be used to determine the locations of specific antigenic structures in a tissue.

3. Enzymes that catalyze the formation of a microscopically visible product can be coupled to antibodies using bifunctional cross-linking reagents, without destroying the activity of the enzyme or the antibody. For example, horseradish peroxidase coupled to a specific antibody and bound to a specific cell or tissue site will convert added hydrogen peroxide to oxygen free radicals. These radicals in turn react with a chromogenic precursor (3, 3'-diaminobenzidine or 4-chloro-1-naphthol) to form an insoluble colored precipitate (Figure 5–15).

4. Antibodies can be made visible in the electron microscope by coupling to electron-dense or morphologically distinguishable particles. Antibodies coupled to ferritin, an iron storage protein from spleen that consists of a protein shell with a ferric hydroxide core, are seen in the electron microscope as small dense spots (Figure 5–16). Antibodies also can be linked to hemocyanin, a large oxygen-carrying protein complex from crustacean hemo-

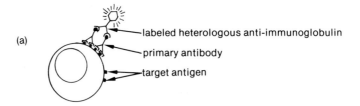

(a)

labeled heterologous anti-immunoglobulin

primary antibody

target antigen

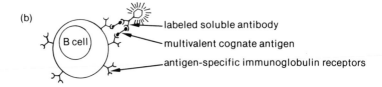

(b)

labeled soluble antibody

multivalent cognate antigen

antigen-specific immunoglobulin receptors

B cell

Figure 5–17   Extension of immunolabeling techniques by (a) the indirect method, and (b) the sandwich method.

lymph, to latex microspheres, or to small viruses, all of which can be visualized by their characteristic morphology in electron micrographs.

5. Each of the preceding four techniques can be extended by a modification called the *indirect method,* which allows detection of unlabeled antibodies bound to a specific antigen by subsequent reaction with a labeled heterologous anti-immunoglobulin (Figure 5–17a). Another modification, called the *sandwich method,* can be used to detect a specific antibody on the surface of plasma cells by incubating them first with a cognate multivalent antigen, and then with labeled soluble antibody specific for the same antigen (Figure 5–17b).

Selected Bibliography

Berson, S. A., and Yalow, R. S., Radioimmunoassay: A status report, in *Immunobiology* (ed. Good, R. A. and Fisher, D. W.), Ch. 30, Sinauer Associates, Inc., Stamford, Conn., 1971. A clear, simple exposition of the principles and practice of radioimmunoassay by its developers.

Eisen, H. N., *Immunology,* Harper and Row, Hagerstown, Md., 1974. A general text that offers a clear explanation of antigen–antibody interaction.

Garvey, J. S., Cremer, N. E., and Sussdorf, D. H., *Methods in Immunology* (3rd edition), Addison-Wesley Publishing Co., Reading, Mass., 1977. This is the third edition of a classic textbook of immunological methods.

Kabat, E. A., *Structural Concepts in Immunology and Immunochemistry* (2nd edition), Holt, Rinehart and Winston, New York, 1976. A thorough monograph for advanced students.

Exercises

5–1   Indicate whether each of the following statements is true or false. Explain the error in each statement you consider to be false.

   T (a)   The lattice formation of antibody–antigen complexes is possible because of the multivalent nature of antibodies and antigens.

   F (b)   The equivalence point of a precipitin curve corresponds to the point at which a maximum antibody–antigen precipitate is obtained.

T   (c)   In the Ouchterlony double-diffusion technique, a reaction of partial identity suggests that the antiserum recognizes at least two distinct antigenic determinants.

T   (d)   The immunoelectrophoresis technique separates individual components of antigenic mixtures by two distinct physical techniques.

F   (e)   A heterologous antiserum is one that is raised in the same species that provided the test antibody.

T   (f)   The ABO blood group antigens are made up of carbohydrate components.

T   (g)   Individuals of the O blood group are universal donors.

5-2   Supply the missing word or words in each of the following statements.

(a)   _Immunoelect_ employs electrophoresis and double diffusion in agar to separate and visualize antigens.

(b)   Immunoglobulins are found in the ___γ___ and ___β___ globulin fractions.

(c)   The ___Farr___ assay employs ammonium sulfate precipitation of immunoglobulins and can be used to measure the concentration of monovalent haptens.

(d)   The association constant of an antibody site for a monovalent hapten can be determined by _equilibrium dialysis_

(e)   The presence or absence of two cell-surface antigens, ___A___ and ___B___, define the four well-known human blood groups: ___AB___, ___A___, ___B___, and ___O___.

(f)   Cellular antigens can be detected directly using specific antibodies with attached _fluores._, _radioisot_, _enzymatic_, or _electron_ markers. _opaque_

Answers are given on page 156.

6 TRANSPLANTATION IMMUNOLOGY

A long-standing goal of physicians and surgeons has been to replace defective organs with functioning transplants from another individual. By the turn of the century surgeons began to recognize that failure of such grafts to "take" was not due to the lack of the surgeon's skill, but represented an active immune response of the host against the transplant. This chapter considers the biological basis of graft rejection, as well as the methods used to suppress the rejection reaction.

Essential Concepts

6-1 Rejection of tissue and organ grafts is due to immunological recognition of cell-surface antigens

A. Grafts from an individual to himself (called *autografts*) almost invariably succeed, and are especially important in treatment of burn patients. Likewise, grafts between two genetically identical individuals (*syngeneic* grafts) almost invariably succeed. However, grafts between two genetically dissimilar individuals of the same species (*allogeneic* grafts), or between individuals of different species (*xenogeneic* grafts), do not succeed. The major reason for their failure is a T-cell-mediated immune response to cell-surface antigens that distinguish donor from host. The tissue antigens that induce an immune response in other individuals are called *histocompatibility antigens,* and the genes that specify their structure and synthesis are called *histocompatibility genes.*

B. In all species tested, there appear to be two categories of histocompatibility genes. The first category, genes of the major histocompatibility complex (MHC), specify antigens that induce rapid rejection of grafts. The second category, termed minor histocompatibility genes, specify antigens that cause a slower graft rejection when acting alone. The MHC is a chromosomal region that comprises a number of closely linked genes which are highly polymorphic within a species, and all of which appear to be involved in immune response and cellular recognition functions. A comparison of the MHC of man and mouse is shown in Figure 6–1.

The T-cell immune response to MHC products in the mouse usually involves recognition of separate MHC products by separate classes of interacting T cells. When lymphocytes from two genetically different individuals of a species are mixed in cell culture medium, the T cells of each individual recognize and respond to MHC antigens presented by cells of the other. In the course of this process, called the *mixed lymphocyte response* (MLR), small T_A cells react first, by enlarging, dividing, releasing lymphokines, and stimulating maturation of T_C effector cells. T_A cells generally respond to Ia antigens on macrophages and B cells more than to antigens coded by the D or K regions (Figure 6–1). Conversely, T_C cells generally recognize and respond to D/K antigens more than to Ia antigens. This distinction may be analogous to the differing recognition specificities of T_H and B cells in the humoral response to a hapten-carrier antigen (Essential Concept 4–4). In both responses T_H category helper cells recognize one set of determinants (Ia antigens or carrier) and stimulate mature T_C or B cells, which recognize a second set of associated determinants (D/K antigens or haptens) and differentiate to effector cytotoxic T_C cells and Ig-secreting plasma cells, respectively (Essential Concept 4–7).

T_C-cell responses to *minor* histocompatibility antigens involve a complex recognition of the minor antigen and self D/K specificities. This is termed associated recognition, to signify that simultaneous recognition of major and minor histocompatibility antigens is required for rejection by T_C cells (Essential Concept 4–7).

C.   The analysis of histocompatibility genetics in mice required the development of inbred strains by repeated brother-sister mating through

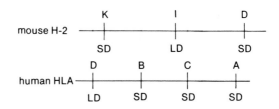

Figure 6–1 Arrangement of subloci in the MHC complexes of mouse and man. In both species antigens specified by the MHC have been identified as serologically defined (SD) antigens (K and D antigens in mouse; B, C, and A antigens in human), or as lymphocyte-defined (LD) antigens (I in mouse; D in human). The SD antigens are found on almost all cells, whereas the LD antigens are present only in some tissues.

20 or more generations. Within such an inbred strain, all mice are virtually identical genetically except for sex. Thus there is MHC (and minor H-gene) identity *within* a strain, and due to the high degree of polymorphism, MHC nonidentity *between* most strains. In mice, the MHC was the second histocompatibility locus named, and is therefore called the H-2 complex. Each H-2 haplotype (combination of distinct genes within the MHC) is named by a letter (e.g., $H-2^a$, $H-2^b$), and the genetic designation of inbred strains accordingly is $H-2^{a/a}$, $H-2^{b/b}$, and so on.

D.   If two strains of mice differ only in the H-2 regions (e.g., $H-2^{a/a}$ and $H-2^{b/b}$), F_1 progeny of an intercross ($H-2^{a/b}$) will accept grafts from either parental strain, but either parental strain will reject grafts from an F_1 donor (Figure 6–2). Thus MHC genes are expressed codominantly. If F_1's are intercrossed to obtain an F_2 generation, three-fourths of the offspring will accept grafts from either one of the original

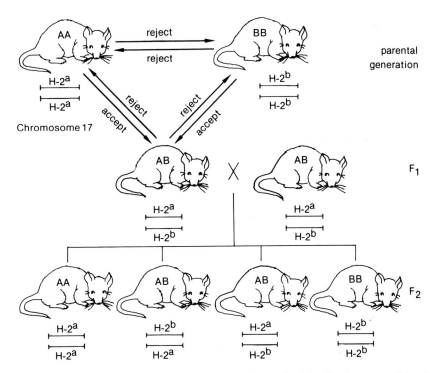

Figure 6–2   Genetics of histocompatibility antigens in inbred mice. Each inbred mouse strain is homozygous for the H-2 complex (e.g., $H-2^a$ or $H-2^b$). Both sets of products are expressed in the heterozygous F_1 hybrids. These mice therefore produce H-2 antigens that stimulate an immune response in either parental strain, whereas neither parental strain expresses H-2 antigens foreign to the F_1 hybrid. In the F_2 generation there is a classical Mendelian 1:2:1 distribution of homozygous and heterozygous genotypes.

parent strains, and half will accept grafts from both. In general, the probability of graft acceptance from parent to F_2 in crosses between inbred strains of mice is $(3/4)^n$, in which n = the number of distinct histocompatibility differences between the two strains. In the preceding simplified example, H-2 acts as a single histocompatibility difference. In reality, for two inbred strains chosen at random, $n \geq 30$. Thus there are at least 29 distinct minor H-loci.

E.   Humans are an outbred species, and thus almost always will be heterozygous at MHC loci. This fact is critical in the choice of a donor for organ or tissue transplants. Mild immunosuppression allows long-term retention of grafts between individuals differing only at minor H-loci, but is insufficient when an MHC difference is involved. Figure 6–3 illustrates the situation in humans. All grafts between parents, from either parent to children, or from children to parents will involve at least one MHC incompatibility. Sibling grafts have a 25% chance of MHC compatibility.

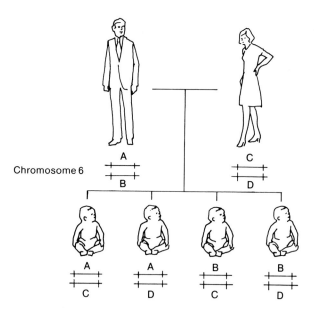

Figure 6–3 Genetics of human histocompatibility antigens. Since humans are not inbred, and the HLA system is highly polymorphic, it is likely that any two parents will possess four distinct MHC haplotypes (e.g., A/B, C/D). The F_1 progeny of such a cross will express four distinct haplotype groups: A/C, A/D, B/C, and B/D. Each parent will express one HLA haplotype foreign to each child, and thus parental grafts are rejected by F_1 progeny. Each child will express one HLA haplotype foreign to each parent, and thus F_1 grafts are rejected by parents. On the average, one in four grafts exchanged between F_1 individuals will be histocompatible at the HLA locus.

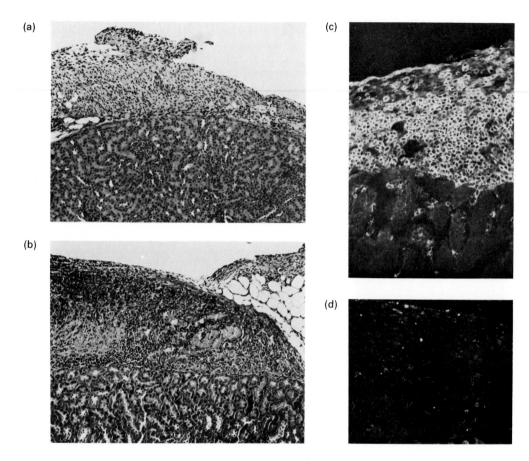

Figure 6–4 A slice of heart tissue from strain C mouse was transplanted under the kidney capsule of another strain C mouse (a), or a strain B mouse (b), 6 days before these sections of tissue were removed for analysis. In (a) the pale tissue on top is heart muscle, and the dark spots are cardiac muscle nuclei. The darker tissue below is normal kidney tissue. In (b) the pale appearance of heart muscle is obscured by the infiltration of many small, dark spots. These are lymphocytes and macrophages. An anti-T-cell stain of another section from (b) is shown in panel (c), demonstrating that a high proportion of the infiltrating cells are T lymphocytes. An anti-B-cell stain is used in (d), demonstrating that B cells are rare or nonexistent in the lymphoid infiltrate. By 12 days after grafting, all allogeneic grafts have disappeared and all syngeneic grafts are retained. [Photographs by M. Billingham, R. Warnke, and I. Weissman.]

6–2   Both T- and B-cell systems may be active in graft rejection

Most graft-rejection reactions are T-cell mediated (Figure 6–4). However, humoral antibodies also can effect rejection in certain cases. The primacy of cellular immunity in graft rejection first was established with skin and tumor grafts. Skin and tumor cells are relatively resistant to antibody-mediated damage, but are susceptible to cell-mediated damage.

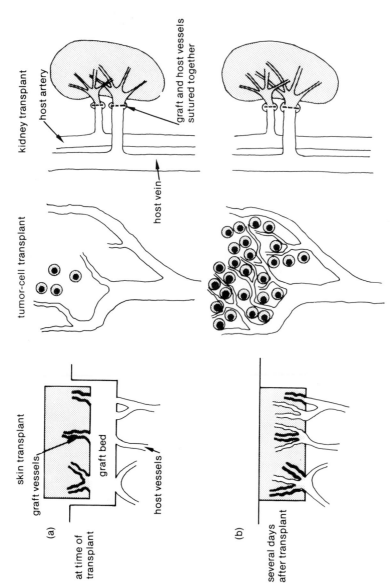

Figure 6–5   The vascular supply of various transplants. (a) At the time of transplantation, only organ grafts (e.g., kidneys) that have the blood vessels surgically joined have an immediate blood supply and therefore do *not* release stimuli for host vessel proliferation and revascularization of donor cells. Both skin grafts and tumor cells induce the release of angiogenic (blood-vessel inducing) factors. (b) Host vessel proliferation may result in the setting up of new channels, or in the natural anastomosis (joining) of host and donor vessels.

However, with the advent of organ grafting in man, a new form of antibody-mediated graft rejection occasionally has been found to occur. The reason for this so-called "hyperacute" rejection is illustrated in Figure 6–5. Whereas revascularization of skin and tumor grafts involves host blood vessels, the vascularization of an organ graft is entirely donor in origin. Therefore, in organ grafts anti-MHC antibodies encounter donor MHC antigens on endothelial cells of vessel linings. These cells are susceptible to antibody-mediated damage, presumably via complement activation and antibody-dependent cell-mediated cytotoxicity. Complement components are consumed and localized to vascular endothelial cells of the graft. The resulting combined cytotoxic and acute inflammatory reaction shuts off blood supply to the organ graft, causing graft death.

1.   Production of high concentrations of anti-donor-MHC antibodies in these cases occurs usually for one of three reasons: insufficient immunosuppression in the grafted host, rejection of a prior transplant that shared some MHC determinants with the new transplant, or immunization with leukocytes that carried cross-reacting MHC antigens. Such leukocytes may have been introduced by previous blood transfusions.

2.   In the latter two cases, pre-existing antibodies may act on the new graft as it is being sutured into place, which results in so-called hyperacute rejection. The grafted organ turns gray due to anoxia, and histological examination of the graft vessels demonstrates massive accumulation of polymorphonuclear leukocytes and blood clotting. In addition, immunofluorescence analysis demonstrates immunoglobulin and complement bound to vessels.

3.   Although antibodies to MHC determinants may cause "hyperacute" rejection of organ allografts, such antibodies may act in different circumstances to interfere with T-cell immunity. This phenomenon, called *immunological enhancement,* is covered in more detail in Chapter 8.

6–3   Three methods of immunosuppression can be used to permit allogeneic graft survival

A.   Nonspecific immunosuppression of the host with antimitotic agents, adrenal steroids, and antilymphocyte sera permits long-term survival of most MHC-matched allografts, and of about 25% of allografts that differ in MHC determinants. However, such immunosuppressed patients are all immunodeficient, and a significant proportion of them suffer life-threatening infections. Even anti-T-cell sera are relatively

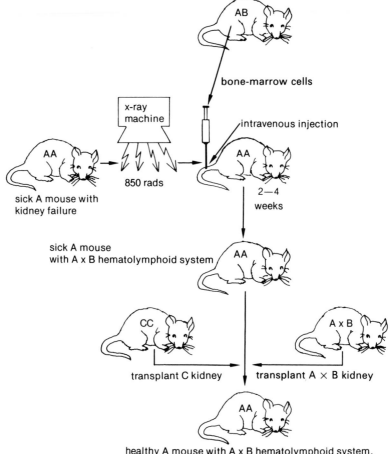

Figure 6–6 Strategy for replacement of the host hematolymphoid system, and subsequent successful allogeneic graft transplantation (see text).

nonspecific, in that all T cells are susceptible, even to the most highly purified antiserum. Because most sera are not highly purified, other cell and tissue systems are at risk as well.

B. Replacement of the host hematolymphoid system by donor bone-marrow cells after host marrow has been eliminated by x-radiation permits subsequent successful allogeneic transplantation of donor grafts. As shown in Figure 6–6, an A mouse that has been given an (A × B)F$_1$ hematopoietic and lymphoid system in this manner accepts an (A × B)F$_1$ (or even a B) kidney graft but rejects a kidney graft from strain C. If strain B bone-marrow cells had been injected following irradiation, subsequent B kidney grafts also would have been accepted. However, the grafted marrow invariably contains a few T cells, some of which recognize and respond to A-strain MHC antigens. The result is a multisystem graft-versus-host response (GVHR), which causes T-cell injury to all organs and usually is fatal. The nature of MHC differences in the outbred human population and the dangers of extensive irradiation do not permit this type of marrow transplant in humans. Elimination of donor-marrow T lymphocytes and their precursors is not feasible at this time.

C.   Transplantation tolerance has been created in rodents by transfusion of $(A \times B)F_1$ spleen or bone-marrow cells into fetal or neonatal A hosts. In this procedure, tolerance presumably results from clonal abortion, although other mechanisms, including suppression by T_S cells, have been suggested. This procedure works only in animals that are accessible for transfusion before the full onset of immune competence. Humans probably have passed that stage by the end of the second trimester of gestation, long before organ failure and the need for transplantation have become apparent. In addition, if a host is sufficiently immature immunologically to accept the donor cellular antigens intended to induce tolerance, then the host also cannot reject donor T cells that are reactive to host MHC antigens. Thus, following such a transfusion a lethal GVHR will ensue unless the tolerance-inducing donor inoculum were genetically (as with inbred rodents) or immunologically unable to respond to host MHC antigens.

D.   Despite these problems, modern immunological approaches eventually may lead to a safe method of allotransplantation. The goal of these approaches is to selectively remove or inactivate clones of host T cells that recognize donor MHC antigens, leaving the rest of the T-cell repertoire intact. Two current and promising approaches are development of specific anti-T-cell-receptor sera, and isolation of MHC antigens in order to make them tolerance-inducing, for example, by changing their form or by coupling them to D-polypeptides for T-cell receptor blockade. See p. 63.

Selected Bibliography

Bach, F. H., and van Rood, J. J., "The major histocompatibility complex—genetics and biology," *N.E.J.M.* **295**, 806–892, 927 (1976). A major review of current knowledge of the genetics of transplantation.

Billingham, R., and Silvers, W., *The Immunobiology of Transplantation,* Prentice-Hall Inc., Englewood Cliffs, N.J., 1971. A short, lucid presentation of the biology of tissue and organ transplantation.

Exercises

6–1   Indicate whether each of the following statements is true or false. Explain the error in each statement you consider to be false.

F   (a)   Allogeneic kidney transplants between identical twins require long-term immunosuppression with adrenal steroids.

T   (b)   Parent-to-offspring transplants are accepted in inbred laboratory mice but are rejected in humans.

F   (c)   Allogeneic skin transplants are more susceptible to antibody-mediated rejection than are mismatched blood transfusions.

F   (d)   A breakdown of the placental barrier to transfer of maternal lymphocytes into a first trimester fetus is of no consequence to the fetus, which will reject the maternal cells as foreign.

T   (e)   Current successful techniques for establishing immunological tolerance to tissue transplants in laboratory animals cannot yet be applied successfully to humans.

6–2   Supply the missing word or words in each of the following statements.

(a)   Hyperacute rejection of organ allografts involves infiltration of _PMNs_.

(b)   Rejection of allogeneic skin transplants involves infiltration of _lymphs_ and _macrophages_.

(c)   The major human MHC product recognized by allogeneic lymphocytes in the mixed lymphocyte response are _HLA-D_ determinants, whereas cytotoxic Tc cells recognize primarily _HLA-A_, _HLA-B_, and _HLA-C_ determinants.

(d)   The current method of prolonging graft survival in humans has as an undesirable side effect nonspecific _immunodef_, which results in a high incidence of _infection_.

Answers are given on pages 156–157.

7 IMMUNOPATHOLOGY

Diseases of the immune system can be grouped into two general classes. *Deficiency* diseases result when a component of the system fails to function. These diseases all manifest themselves clinically by low resistance to infection and loss of other immunologic surveillance functions. *Hypersensitivity* diseases result when the system reacts under inappropriate conditions. These diseases lead to a variety of pathologic symptoms. Some diseases of both classes are congenital, whereas others are acquired. This chapter considers the causes and consequences of immune deficiency and hypersensitivity. The first half deals primarily with the cellular or molecular bases of deficiency diseases. The second half describes the inappropriate responses of T cells and B cells in hypersensitivity diseases, and concludes by returning to a recurrent theme in modern immunology: the role of gene products coded by the major histocompatibility complex in normal and pathological immune responses.

Essential Concepts

7-1 Lowered resistance to infection may result from defects in general host defenses

Immunity to infection depends upon a combination of nonspecific innate functions and specific T- and B-cell adaptive immune responses. The nonspecific functions prevent invasion by the vast majority of microorganisms. Some of the most important of these functions are: maintenance of epithelial surface integrity; action of antibacterial substances such as lysozyme (an enzyme in secretions that attacks bacterial cell walls) and C-reactive protein (an inducible serum factor that binds to bacterial cell-wall phosphorylcholine residues and activates complement-mediated opsonization and lysis); maintenance of local pH conditions, for example acidity in the stomach and vagina; and mechanical expulsion of microorganisms by various mechanisms such as ciliary movement on respiratory tract epithelium and the sneeze reflex. Failure of any of these innate defenses may lead to infection in the absence of any immunologic deficiency disease.

If microorganisms successfully invade epithelial barriers, most of them are removed by the phagocytic system, which also stimulates the specific functions of T- and B-cell immunity. Because most immunologic reactions also end with phagocytosis and degradation of the antigenic microorganisms, it is appropriate to begin the discussion of lymphoid system deficiencies with malfunctions of phagocytic cells.

7-2   Diseases that interfere with phagocytic functions usually result in lethal bacterial infections

A.   The elimination of invading microorganisms by phagocytic cells is a multistep process. It includes chemotactic attraction of phagocytes to the site of infection, phagocytosis of invading microorganisms, intracellular union of phagosomes and lysosomes, and lysosomal destructive action involving enzymatic iodination of microorganism cell walls leading to their breakdown by various acidic hydrolases. In normal hosts most types of microorganisms are eliminated by this process. Consequently these microorganisms are nonpathogenic (not disease generating). A few types of microorganisms regularly survive these events, and hence are pathogenic.

Patients with malfunctioning phagocytic cells have recurrent infections, usually caused by normally nonpathogenic organisms, which become pathogenic in these hosts. Such phagocytic malfunction diseases are relatively rare, and usually are inherited. Practical diagnosis of these disorders involves isolation and testing of blood phagocytes for (a) motile responses to chemotactic factors, (b) ability to phagocytize a range of microorganisms, (c) ability to kill phagocytosed microorganisms, and (d) ability to generate hydrogen peroxide, H_2O_2, which is required in the iodinations of microorganisms, and can be measured *in vitro* using the redox-sensitive dye, nitroblue tetrazolium.

B.   Two forms of phagocytic-cell disease have been described in humans.

1.   One of these diseases involves a defect of lysosomal structure in phagocytes and other cells. These cells have abnormally large lysosomes that lyse bacteria ineffectively, and fuse sluggishly with phagosomes, although phagocytosis is normal. Humans with this disease, called *Chediak-Higashi syndrome,* are also partial albinos, presumably due to a related defect of structures similar to lysosomes in the pigmented cells of the retina and skin. The disease usually is fatal in childhood. Related disorders have been found in mink (Aleutian mink disease), cattle, and mice.

2.   A second form of phagocytic malfunction is due to defects in the lysosomal enzymes that produce H_2O_2, or those that act on H_2O_2 to produce oxygen-free radicals required in the iodination of microorganisms. Cells from patients with this disease phagocytize, but do not kill most bacteria, which continue to grow inside the phagocytes and induce a prolonged local inflammatory reaction. The combination of activated phagocytes and surrounding cells growing in a nodule is identifiable histologically as a *granuloma.* Such granulomatous diseases usually are fatal in childhood, and can exhibit either of two modes of inheritance: an X-linked recessive form known as *chronic granulomatous disease,* and an autosomal recessive form known as *Job's syndrome* (Figure 7–1a).

7–3   Some patients lack both T- and B-cell systems

Congenital lack of lymphocytes, known as *severe combined immunodeficiency,* may result from any one of several defects. Three distinct genetic bases for these diseases are known: an X-linked recessive, an autosomal recessive defect of the enzyme *adenosine deaminase,* and an autosomal recessive of unknown primary effect. How or why each of these defects eliminates only the lymphoid compartment of the hematolymphoid system is unknown.

Patients with these defects are extraordinarily susceptible to microorganisms that grow either inside host cells—mainly viruses and a few types of bacteria—or outside host cells—mainly bacteria. These patients lack a lymphoid thymus, and their blood, spleen, lymph nodes, Peyers patches, tonsils, and appendix also lack lymphocytes. They have no serum immunoglobulins. In some patients, bone-marrow cell transplants may completely repopulate both T- and B-cell systems. Because both T and B cells but no other blood cell types are missing in these patients, the defects apparently are at the level of cells that are committed to lymphoid maturation, but are not yet committed to either T- or B-cell lineages (Figure 7–1b).

7–4   Some patients lack only the T-cell system

A.   Individuals who lack T cells are especially susceptible to viral and bacterial intracellular infections. Vaccination of these individuals with live, attenuated (normally nonpathogenic) viruses usually is fatal. In general, T cells are absent from their blood and lymphoid tissues,

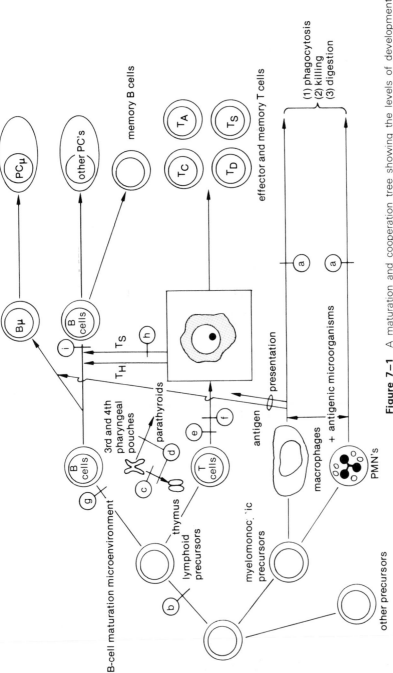

Figure 7–1 A maturation and cooperation tree showing the levels of developmental defects that result in cellular immunological deficiency diseases. (a) Defects in phagocytic function, seen in Chediak–Higashi syndrome, Job's syndrome, and fatal granulomatous disease. (b) Presumed block in severe combined immunodeficiency syndromes. (c) Thymic dysplasia. (d) DiGeorge syndrome. (e) Episodic lymphopenia with lymphocytotoxins. (f) Hodgkin's disease. (g) Bruton's disease. (h) Acquired hypogammaglobulinemia with suppressor cells. (i) Selective dysgammaglobulinemias. Abbreviations: HSC, hematopoietic stem cell; T, T cell; B, B cell; PMN, polymorphonuclear leukocyte; PC, plasma cell.

and they lack testable T-cell functions, such as graft rejection and activation of blood lymphocytes in response to the T-cell mitogenic (mito: division, genic: capable of causing) lectins concanavalin A and phytohemagglutinin.

B.   Several congenital defects can lead to specific lack of T cells.

1.   One such defect, characterized by disorganized tissue in the thymus, is known as *thymic dysplasia* (Figure 7–1c).

2.   A second defect is characterized by lack of the thymic (and parathyroid) inductive microenvironment, presumably a result of improper formation of the third and fourth pharyngeal endodermal pouches during embryogenesis (Figure 7–1d). This congential abnormality, known as the *DiGeorge syndrome,* is not heritable. Children with this abnormality can be recognized clinically because they also lack parathyroid hormones and therefore cannot maintain appropriate calcium levels in the blood. Consequently, soon after birth they go into muscle spasm (hypocalcemic tetany).

C.   Some *acquired* diseases also result in a total or partial lack of peripheral T cells.

1.   Some patients show episodic decreases in T cells, accompanied by the expected range of immunodeficiencies. During these episodes the patients produce a serum autoantibody that lyses T cells in the presence of complement. This disease is known as *episodic lymphopenia with lymphocytotoxins* (Figure 7–1e).

2.   An acquired T-cell deficiency also occurs in patients with *Hodgkin's disease,* a cancer of lymph-node cells. Although the malignant cells may be limited to a single lymph node, these patients exhibit a whole-body deficiency of T-cell functions: for example, delayed allograft rejection, weak contact sensitivity, and decreased resistance to intracellular infections such as tuberculosis and Herpes viruses. These patients have normal numbers of peripheral T cells as measured by anti-T-cell antisera, but these cells respond weakly to T-cell mitogens, and do not exhibit the normal ability to bind sheep red blood cells nonspecifically. The surface receptors of T cells from these patients appear to be blocked by serum factors that are elevated markedly in Hodgkin's disease (Figure 7–1f).

7–5   Some patients lack only the B-cell system

A.   A total congenital lack of B cells, their progeny and their products, can result from another X-linked recessive gene defect. Patients with this syndrome, called *infantile sex-linked agammaglobulinemia* or *Bruton's disease* (Figure 7–1g), are especially susceptible to pyogenic (pus-causing) bacterial infections of the skin and respiratory tracts, beginning at about six months of age, when placentally transferred maternal immunoglobulin has disappeared. The lives of these patients can be saved by inoculation with gamma globulin pooled from several different donors, which usually prevents infections.

B.   Several *acquired* B-cell defects also are known. These diseases, all poorly understood, include both complete and partial defects of B cells and their immunoglobulin products.

   1.   One class of patients with *acquired agammaglobulinemia* has normal levels of B cells, but no plasma cells (Figure 7–1h). *In vitro* analysis has demonstrated that these patients possess a class of T_S cells that prevents stimulation of antibody formation. Thus this disease may be classified more properly as a T-cell abnormality.

   2.   Selective deficiencies of IgA, or IgA and IgG, often are associated with gastrointestinal tract disorders, such as diarrhea and poor intestinal absorption of fats and fat-soluble vitamins, by mechanisms that are not understood. Patients with these deficiencies have normal numbers of B_α cells, and these cells can be stimulated to become IgA-secreting plasma cells *in vitro* (Figure 7–1i). Several other such *selective dysgammaglobulinemias* (dysfunctions of particular immunoglobulin classes in the blood) have been reported, including deficiencies in IgM alone, IgM and IgA, or IgM and IgG. Deficiencies in IgM and IgG usually are accompanied by susceptibility to pyogenic infections.

7-6   Some immune deficiencies are secondary to other diseases, or are unexplained

A.   Immunological deficiency may be secondary to diseases which result in the accumulation of immunosuppressive products. For example, defective function of the kidney or liver leads to an accumulation of toxic substances which may depress immune responses. Patients ill with virus infections often release immunosuppressive products into the blood, as do many patients with advanced cancers.

   A well-known multisystem disease that leads to a deficiency in immunity is called *Cushing's disease.* It is caused by the excess secretion of cortisone and cortisol, two hormones of the adrenal cortex. These hormones have several effects at these increased concentrations: potent anti-inflammatory actions, direct lysis of most T and B cells, and decreased levels of blood monocytes. Patients with Cushing's disease become extremely susceptible to infection, particularly to those agents usually controlled by the T-cell system. The increased secretion of the two hormones may be episodic, related to periods of emotional or physical stress.

B.   Because the immune system employs cellular biochemical mechanisms common to several other cell systems, it frequently may be affected by defects in these mechanisms. Such a defect may first become apparent clinically as failure of immunity, leading to early infection, and careful analysis may be required to show that the defect in fact is more general.

   1.   *Adenosine deaminase deficiency* is one example of a general defect that is manifested most clearly as an immune-system abnormality. Patients who are deficient in this enzyme, usually present in tissues and red cells, lack both T and B cells.

   2.   Patients with *ataxia-telangiectasia* are defective in their ability to repair x-ray-induced damage to DNA. In early life their immune system appears normal. As they grow older, they develop pathological alterations in their small veins with the formation of *telangiectases* (*tel*: end; *angio*: vessel; *ectases*: stretching out), which are highly dilated, tortuous venous networks. These alterations first become apparent as effects on the cerebellum, resulting in disorders of balance and movement (ataxia). Later, telangiectases become visible in the skin and the whites of the eyes. Beginning in about the fifth year of life, these patients develop a progressive immune deficiency that is characterized by defective cellular immunity and, often, by a total lack of IgA (and sometimes IgE). The thymus is alymphoid in these patients by the time the immunological defects appear. No clear relationship between the x-ray sensitivity of the cells from these patients and their subsequent pathology has yet been established.

   3.   Another unexplained, multisystem, progressive disease that results in the loss of T cells is called *Wiskott–Aldrich syndrome,* or *immunodeficiency with thrombocytopenia and eczema.* "Thrombocytopenia" means lack of platelets, and eczema is a skin disorder characterized by an inappropriate response of the IgE system to antigens. Patients with this disease are born normal, but at an early age they have problems of bleeding due to lack of platelets, which are important in the blood clotting process. They develop eczematous skin rashes and later show a progressive loss of T-cell functions. The underlying pathological process that causes this distinctive combination of immunodeficiency, thrombocytopenia, and eczema is unknown.

7-7   Most immunological deficiencies result from medical therapy for other diseases

Many therapeutic treatments involve suppression of the immune system, either intentionally or inadvertently. These treatments may have dangerous side effects related to the resulting immunodeficiency. Diseases *caused* by medical therapy are called *iatrogenic* diseases.

1. The potent anti-inflammatory effect of the adrenocortical hormones, cortisone and cortisol, and of their inducer, ACTH (*a*drenoc*o*rtico*t*ropic *h*ormone), has led to widespread use of these agents in the control of diseases that have a major inflammatory component. Prolonged use of these hormones has the same effects as Cushing's disease, and may make infections fatal.

2. Chemotherapy and x-ray therapy of most cancers involve the use of agents that inactivate dividing cells. Because cell division is necessary to generate most effector cells of the immune system, the prolonged use of anticancer agents depletes cells important for host immunity.

3. Transplantation operations to replace defective organs often introduce foreign antigenic tissue into the recipient. Adrenocortical hormones and anticancer drugs, as well as antisera against lymphocytes of the T-cell series, are all used to suppress the host rejection reaction. All these agents cause nonspecific immunosuppression that leads to immunodeficiency.

7-8   Hereditary deficiency of complement system components may be either fatal or trivial

1. Hereditary deficiencies of several complement components involved in acute inflammation (Essential Concept 4–3 D) are known. These deficiencies often, but not invariably, are associated with a decreased resistance to bacterial infections, or an increased incidence of hypersensitivity diseases. Deficiencies of other

Table 7–1

Complement deficiency and associated diseases in man

Deficient component	Associated diseases
Clr	Infections
	Hypersensitivity diseases
Cls	Hypersensitivity diseases
C2	Hypersensitivity diseases, infections
C3	Infections
C4	Hypersensitivity diseases
C5	Infections

complement components usually are not associated with decreased host immunity (Table 7–1).

2. Deficiency of a control element in complement activation, C-1 esterase inhibitor, leads to a condition known as *hereditary angioneurotic edema.* It is believed that normally the complement system may be activated and deactivated repeatedly, but that in patients with this condition the reactions go unchecked, thereby causing recurrent episodes of local acute inflammation at sites of activation. The results are vessel dilation and transudation of fluid into the tissue spaces in the upper respiratory tract, gastrointestinal tract, and skin. If activation occurs in the throat at or near the larynx, it may cause death by suffocation.

7-9 Abnormal autoimmune responses can cause disease

A.   Immune responses to self-components (autoimmune responses) usually do not occur. When they do, some autoimmune responses are pathogenic, whereas others are not. It seems probable that only some components of an immune response to self can cause disease.

B.   Autoimmune responses that represent a failure of immunological tolerance may occur in three ways. *Induction* of tolerance may be interrupted, resulting in the emergence of "forbidden clones" of T and B cells that bear receptors for self-antigens. Since the maturation of lymphocytes occurs continuously, a constant supply of autoantigen must be present to induce tolerance in newly arising virgin lymphocytes. If an autoantigen is not present for an extended period, then breakdown of tolerance will ensue. For example, removal of the pituitary from larval tree frogs results in rejection of the same pituitary when it is reimplanted into the same frog as an adult.

1. The failure of antigen-specific suppression by T_S cells may allow clones of antiself-lymphocytes to be activated. Loss of specific T_S cells or nonspecific loss of this class of cells could result in the spontaneous appearance of autoantibodies.

2. An immune response to nonself-antigens may activate lymphocytes that bear antiself-receptors and had formerly been maintained in a state of nonreactivity. Low zone tolerance may involve tolerance at the T-cell but not the B-cell level (Essential Concept 4–9C). Therefore, if some breakdown of T-cell tolerance occurs, *humoral* autoimmunity may result from presentation of autoantigens to clones of B antiself-cells via the newly activated T_H cells.

Three models of how such an event may occur are shown in Figure 7–2. Panel (a) shows the normal tolerant response to

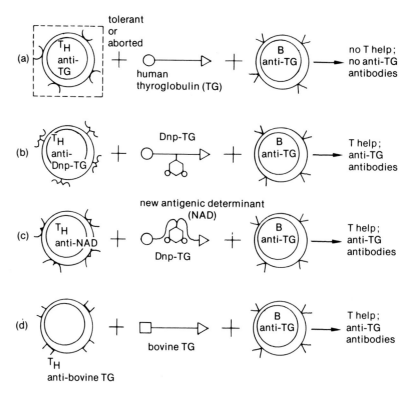

Figure 7–2 Mechanisms by which tolerance to an autologous thyroglobulin (TG) may be broken. (a) Normal tolerance; lack of active T_H anti-TG cells prevents triggering of B anti-TG cells. Hapten modification of TG by Dnp, for example, can result in stimulation of T_H cells which react to either (b) Dnp–TG or (c) new antigenic determinants (NAD) revealed on the hapten-modified TG. (d) Injection of TG from another species, bovine TG, for example, may stimulate T_H cells reactive to bovine-TG specific antigenic determinants.

an autologous thyroid protein, thyroglobulin (TG). Panels (b) and (c) show possible consequences of modifying thyroglobulin by combination with Dnp to produce a Dnp-TG conjugate. The Dnp itself may provide an antigenic determinant recognizable by clones of anti-Dnp-TG T_H cells (Panel b), or the Dnp may lead to a conformational change in the TG protein that exposes groups that previously were hidden (Panel c). Such groups would constitute *new antigenic determinants* (NAD) to the immune system, and could be recognized by clones of anti-NAD T_H cells. As shown in Panel (d), injection of TG from another species that has cross-reacting as well as unique antigenic determinants may stimulate T_H clones specific for the unique determinants. As in the situation illustrated by Panels (b) and (c), T_H–B

cooperation occurs, and autoantibodies are induced. Once induced, the humoral autoantibodies to TG may eliminate all
circulating TG, theoretically permitting the emergence of both
T- and B-cell clones that are reactive to self TG.

The example in Panel (d) is potentially relevant to patients
who receive animal-hormone replacement therapy, for example
with bovine insulin or ACTH. A similar situation probably occurs
in *rheumatic fever*, in which certain streptococci carry antigenic
determinants that cross-react with heart muscle. A similar situation probably also gives rise to the brain and nerve damage that
can follow a rabies vaccination if the rabies vaccine is prepared
from heterologous brain tissue.

7-10 The T-cell system may react inappropriately to cause disease

Inappropriate T-cell immunity can be defined as a state in which activated
T cells initiate or promote disease. This state may come about through
immunity to microorganisms, immunity to haptens that couple to
endogenous proteins, or immunity to endogenous antigens themselves.

1. An example of immunopathogenic T-cell immunity to microorganisms is the neurological disease induced by the lymphocytic
choriomeningitis virus (LCM). This virus infects the choroid
membrane of the third and fourth lateral ventricles of the brain
and the membranous meninges that cover the brain, inducing
infiltration of lymphocytes into these tissues. The neurological
damage is not caused by the virus itself, but by the T-cell-
dependent cellular immune response to the virus-infected cells.
Evidence for this conclusion is that the viral infection is not
lethal in thymectomized hosts. Thus a specific T-cell immune
response may destroy vital cells and cause disease.

2. T-cell immunity to a microorganism can cause disease if
the immune response does not eliminate the microorganism.
Tuberculosis provides a good example of this process. The
tubercle bacillus primarily infects host macrophages. During its
intracellular life it is unaffected by humoral immunity. Most types
of tubercle bacilli are killed within activated macrophages, as
a result of macrophage interaction with T cells immune to the
tubercle bacillus. However, a few resistant strains of tubercle
bacilli can proliferate within macrophages in the face of an active
and specific T-cell immune response (Figure 7–3a). It has been
reported that these pathogenic mycobacteria release substances
that prevent fusion of phagosomes with lysosomes. Activated
macrophages that carry proliferating tubercle bacilli sometimes

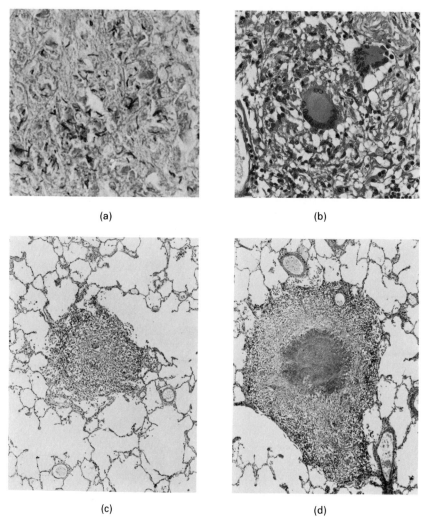

(a)   (b)

(c)   (d)

Figure 7–3   The histological appearance of tuberculosis in the lung. (a) A high-power view of tubercle bacilli inside macrophages, using a dye that stains the rodlike bacilli. (b) A high-power view of cells in an early granuloma. The large multinucleate cells are characteristic of this process. Most of the dark nuclei are lymphocytic; other cells include macrophages and cells involved in repair and regeneration. (c) A low-power view of a central granuloma surrounded by relatively normal lung tissue (large air sacs separated by lacy-thin alveolar walls). The granuloma contains a central zone of giant cells and fibrous tissue, with a shell of lymphocytic infiltrate. (d) A higher-power view of a granuloma containing a core of dead tissue and surrounding fibrous tissue, giant cells, and a shell of lymphocytic infiltrate. [Photographs by R. Rouse and I. Weissman.]

are termed epitheloid, because they may assume an abnormal shape resembling that of an epithelial cell. These macrophages also may fuse to form giant syncytial cells (Figure 7–3b).

The result of these conditions is a continuing stimulus for chronic inflammation, with the buildup of a granuloma (Essential Concept 7–2B) of increasing size (Figure 7–3c). As the granuloma enlarges, the signals for repair, which normally accompany chronic inflammation, cause proliferation of fibroblasts at the outer margins of the granuloma, with formation of fibrous tissue. Cells in the central core of the granuloma begin to die (Figure 7–3d), probably due to lack of oxygen, continued proliferation of tubercle bacilli, and release of nonspecific cytotoxins characteristic of chronic inflammation. The central core of dead and dying cells may rupture through the fibrous wall of the granuloma, thereby spreading the live tubercle bacilli to neighboring sites. The granulomas form at the expense of valuable lung tissue, and their rupture has two consequences: it spreads tubercle bacilli, initiating new granulomas, and it forms cavities in the old granulomas, which then cannot be reconverted to functional lung tissue. Thus the T-cell immune response to tubercle bacilli can set in motion a destructive chronic inflammatory granulomatous reaction.

The leprosy bacillus, closely related to the tubercle bacillus, causes a destructive reaction much like that of tuberculosis, following preferential infection of macrophages in the skin and around nerves.

3. T-cell immunity to environmental haptens can cause a local, destructive immune response called *contact sensitivity*. Environmental haptens can bind to protein or cell-membrane carriers in the skin and induce a local T-cell immune reaction to the hapten-conjugated proteins or cells. These haptens can be natural products (e.g., the active small molecules in poison ivy and poison oak leaves), or industrial reagents such as picryl chloride (trinitrophenyl chloride or Tnp), which can form Tnp conjugates via a substitution reaction with the ε-amino groups of lysine. Sufficient concentrations of these *contact sensitizing* agents may induce a T-cell immune response that results in a chronic inflammatory focus as well as direct lysis of hapten-conjugated target cells.

4. T-cell immunity to endogenous antigens can lead to an immunopathologic destruction of vital tissues. The various mechanisms for induction of autoimmunity were described in Essential Concept 7–9. Experimental organ-specific autoimmunity has been demonstrated following the injection of xenogeneic organ homogenates. Such autoimmune reactions have been studied in detail

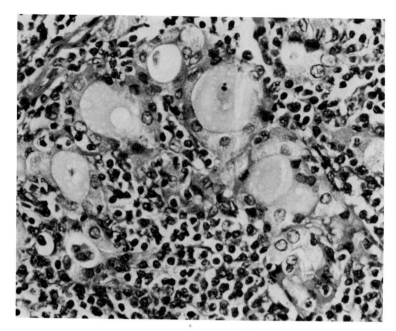

Figure 7–4 Thyroid from a patient with Hashimoto's thyroiditis. The predominant cell types which infiltrate the thyroid are lymphocytes and macrophages. [Photograph by R. Rouse.]

for adrenals (*adrenalitis,* in which the suffix *itis* indicates inflammation of the affected tissue or organ), thyroid (*thyroiditis*), and nervous tissue (*encephalomyelitis*; encephalo: brain, myelo: spinal cord).

Certain human diseases appear to have organ-specific T-cell immunity as a component. For example, in *Hashimoto's thyroiditis,* all patients exhibit a chronic inflammatory reaction in the thyroid, and T cells from some of these patients are reactive to human thyroid antigens (Figure 7–4). In some cases of adrenal insufficiency (*Addison's disease*), cellular autoimmunity to adrenal cell antigens is present.

5. Both cellular and humoral immunity may be able to cause anemia by an indirect mechanism. Some patients with pernicious anemia are unable to absorb vitamin B_{12}, which is necessary for erythroid and myeloid differentiation in the bone marrow. These individuals usually lack intrinsic factor, a polypeptide produced by parietal cells in the stomach, which binds vitamin B_{12} and allows its absorption across the intestinal epithelium. Some of these patients are deficient in parietal cells, presumably as a result of parietal-cell-specific cellular autoimmunity. Others have parietal cells that produce and excrete intrinsic factor, but the factor is neutralized by specific autoantibodies transported to the intestinal lumen.

In general, diseases that have complex, multisystem manifestations that result from loss of an important class of cells may have a T-cell autoimmune origin. A possible example is *juvenile diabetes mellitus,* which is caused by lack of pancreatic islet-of-Langerhans cells. Recent reports indicate that diabetes induced in rats by the drug streptozocin results from the development of cellular immunity to islet cells, probably a consequence of drug-induced damage of these cells.

7-11 Immune complexes of antigen, antibody, and complement can cause local, destructive, inflammatory lesions

A.   Immune complexes (antigen–antibody precipitates) may form in an immune response to a multideterminant antigen if antibody and antigen concentrations are appropriate (Essential Concept 5–1). For antigens confined to lymphoid tissues, complex formation has only minor immunopathological consequences. However, for freely circulating antigens, such as serum proteins, antigen–antibody complexes may be removed both by phagocytic cells and by basement membranes that underlie endothelial cells in blood vessels. Large complexes are phagocytized, whereas smaller complexes may escape phagocytosis and pass between vessel endothelial cells to deposit on subendothelial basement

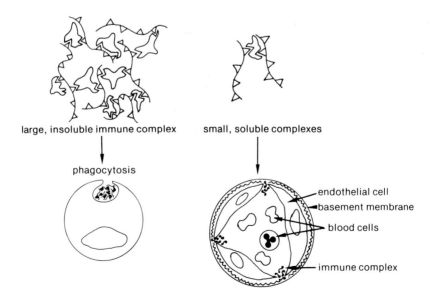

large, insoluble immune complex   small, soluble complexes

phagocytosis

endothelial cell
basement membrane
blood cells
immune complex

Figure 7–5 Fates of large and small complexes of antigen, antibody, and complement (see text).

membranes (Figure 7–5). If these complexes activate complement, they may induce an acute local inflammation at the site of deposition. Usually this effect is transient, as antigen and complexes are cleared and antibody levels rise. However, when the initial antigen load is large the short-term effects may cause serious inflammatory disease. If antigen is reintroduced under these circumstances, chronic or recurrent disease may occur.

1. *Serum sickness* is an example of an immune-complex disease in which the initial antigen load is large. The disease is caused by host immune responses to injected antigenic serum proteins. It was most common in the preantibiotic era, when serum from animals (e.g., horses) immunized against particular pathogenic microorganisms was injected into humans to provide passive immunity to the pathogen or to toxins released by the pathogen.

Figure 7–6 illustrates the course of events in serum sickness following injection of horse immunoglobulin. The levels of horse immunoglobulin at first fall slowly, reflecting the intrinsic degradation rate of these proteins. Beginning at about Day 8, the levels begin to fall more rapidly, as the foreign protein begins to be eliminated by immune complex formation. Concomitant with immune elimination of free horse immunoglobulin is an increase in antigen–antibody complexes, and the appearance of the typical disease pattern: fever, rash, joint lesions, appearance of serum proteins in the urine (proteinuria), and retention in the serum of substances such as urea that normally are cleared by the kidneys. These indications of inflammatory disease subside as immune complexes disappear from the serum and free antibody to horse immunoglobulin appears.

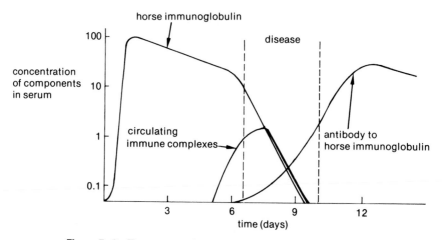

Figure 7–6 Time course of major events in serum sickness (see text).

2. Most, if not all, symptoms of serum sickness are due to activation of the complement system by antigen–antibody complexes. Such activation may cause release of vasoactive (*vaso*: vessel) peptides, which induce vasodilation, thereby revealing larger areas of vascular basement membrane. This process is especially notable in the small capillary tufts of the kidney glomeruli where blood filtration takes place (Figure 7–7). Normally, the kidney glomeruli allow passage of small molecules such as urea, but prevent passage of most serum proteins from the vascular lumen into the space that constitutes the beginning of the urinary tubules (Bowman's space). As immune complexes settle on the epithelial side of the glomerular basement membrane, they continue to activate complement, thereby increasing vasodilation and deposition of immune complexes. These complexes induce release of chemotactic factors that attract polymorphonuclear leukocytes, which tend to disrupt the attachment of epithelial-cell foot processes to the glomerular basement membrane. The leukocytes may degranulate, releasing pyrogens (factors that stimulate brain centers to raise body temperature), and hydrolytic lysosomal enzymes that destroy large areas of the basement membrane. At this stage serum proteins leak into Bowman's space, and the kidney's function of clearing small molecules decreases dramatically. However, as phagocytic cells remove bound immune complexes, cells, and tissue debris, the glomerular endothelial and epithelial cells are replaced by cell division. A similar process occurs in arterioles, where the damage is limited to the inner layers of the arteriolar wall (Figure 7–7b).

3. In serum sickness such immune-complex-mediated local acute inflammation can occur within lymph nodes, to cause swollen glands (lymphadenitis), and in joint spaces, to cause arthritis (*arthro*: joint). The acute inflammation of the glomeruli is called *acute glomerulonephritis.* One type is commonly induced by the immune response to a particular protein (M protein) in streptococci. An acute glomerulonephritis that does *not* involve antibody can occur in blood infections by gram-negative organisms, which activate the alternate complement pathway.

B.   Recurrent or continuous immune-complex disease occurs when the inducing antigens are endogenous, are reinjected, or are produced by infecting organisms that cannot be eliminated.

1. Immune complexes may deposit in skin vessels, to cause local rash and tissue damage (*Arthus phenomenon*), or in systemic blood vessels, to cause *necrotising (necro*: dead or dying) *vasculitis* (*periarteritis nodosa* is an example of a destructive acute inflammatory lesion of small arteries in nodal foci throughout the body).

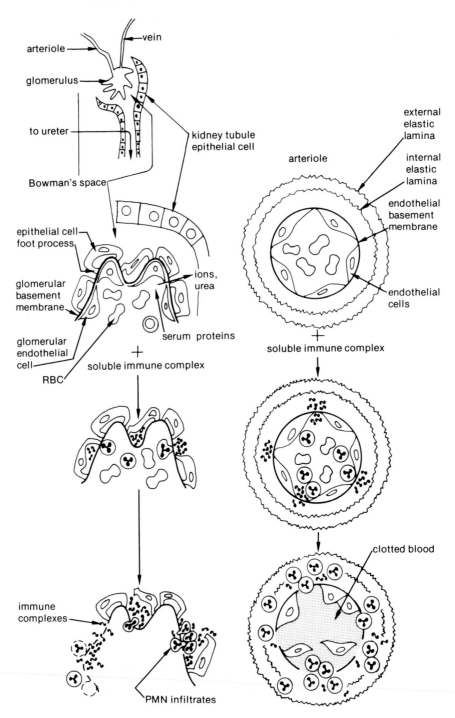

Figure 7–7 (a) Injury to a kidney glomerulus following immune complex deposition. (b) Injury to an arteriole following immune complex deposition (see text).

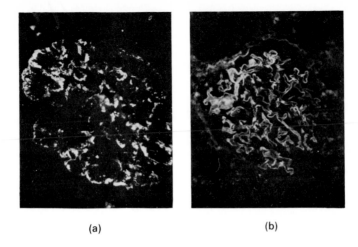

(a)   (b)

Figure 7–8 Immunofluorescence of renal immunoglobulin deposits in glomerulone-phritis. (a) Immune complex nephritis with granular (lumpy-bumpy) deposits of IgG. (b) Good-pasture's syndrome, with linear deposition of IgG on glomerular basement membranes. [Photographs by D. Rice and R. Kempson.]

Immune complexes also may deposit in joints, to cause arthritis. *Rheumatoid arthritis* is a special example in which the antigen may be endogenous IgG, which complexes with circulating IgM antibodies.

2. Some other diseases consist of immune-complex disease in addition to other pathology. For example, *systemic lupus erythematosis* (SLE) is a multisystem autoimmune disorder in which complexes of nucleic acid with specific antibody, or of other tissue components with autoantibody, may affect skin, joints, arteries, muscle, pericardium (tissue surrounding the heart), and glomeruli. The life-threatening immunopathology of SLE usually is either terminal kidney failure or the side effects of immunosuppressive and anti-inflammatory drugs.

C. Immune-complex disease is characterized by granular ("lumpy-bumpy") deposition of immunoglobulin, complement, and antigen on basement membranes underlying the cells that line blood vessels. Because of this characteristic pattern of deposition, immunofluorescence microscopy is often helpful in the diagnosis (Figure 7–8a).

7-12 Antibodies directed against cell-surface or basement-membrane antigens can cause cell death and acute inflammation

Antibodies to cell-surface antigens can cause cell death by direct complement-mediated cytolysis, by antibody-dependent cell-mediated cytotoxicity, and by opsonization. The most common cell types affected are the blood elements—red blood cells (erythrocytes), platelets, poly-morphonuclear leukocytes, and lymphocytes. The cell-surface antigens may be haptens (such as penicillin), alloantigens (on transfused or fetal red blood cells), or autoantigens.

1. If the antigens are on erythrocytes, the usual result is hemolysis (cell lysis that releases free hemoglobin into the serum), and *anemia* (decreased concentration of erythrocytes in the blood). Autoimmune hemolytic anemias often involve hemolysis induced by autoantibodies as well as by antibodies directed against drugs that adsorb to red cells, such as penicillin, quinidine, and α-methyl dopa.

Transfusion of mismatched blood induces formation of antibodies against foreign red blood cell determinants, followed by massive immune hemolysis (*transfusion reaction*). A small transfusion of fetal blood to the mother usually occurs during birth. If an antigen known as Rh is present on fetal blood cells but lacking in the mother, then the mother may produce anti-Rh IgG antibodies. These antibodies can cross the placental barrier and may cause massive antibody destruction of Rh-positive red blood cells in a subsequent fetus (*Erythroblastosis fetalis*). This disease does not occur when there is maternal–fetal incompatibility for the A–B–O blood groups, because all people who lack A or B antigens have significant amounts of "natural" IgM antibodies to the antigens they lack. IgM does not cross the placenta, but will bind to and remove fetal transfusions, thereby preventing the induction of an IgG response.

2. Antibodies to polymorphonuclear leukocytes may be induced by drug treatment: for example, by amidopyrine and sulfa drugs (sulfapyridine, sulfathiazole). The result is *agranulocytosis,* which renders patients highly susceptible to bacterial infections.

3. Autoantibodies to platelets (thrombocytes) may arise after some infections, after some drug therapies, and spontaneously. Such autoantibodies can induce *thrombocytopenic purpura.* The resulting decrease in blood-clotting functions leads to multiple hemorrhages, most visible in the skin and gums as purpura (purple spots). Thrombocytopenic purpura is a general name for platelet-loss diseases, several of which formerly were classed as idiopathic (of unknown origin). Some of these diseases now are known to result from autoimmune responses.

4. Antibodies to vascular basement membranes may cause both complement-mediated lysis and acute inflammation. In a particularly striking form of this condition, called *Goodpasture's syndrome,* autoantibodies are produced against determinants common to glomerular and lung alveolar basement membranes. In the glomerulus, the result is an even, *linear* deposition of immunoglobulin and complement on the endothelial side of the glomerular basement membrane (Figure 7–8b). This deposition may induce infiltration of polymorphonuclear leukocytes and glomerulonephritis. Immunofluorescence microscopy can distinguish this condition from immune-complex glomerulonephritis (Figure 7–8a). Immunopathogenic levels of antibodies to glomerular basement membranes have occurred in kidney transplant patients after kidney rejection, or as a consequence of immunosuppressive treatment with impure antilymphocyte serum (ALS).

7–13   Clinical allergy is caused by an inappropriate IgE response

A.   Some individuals develop exaggerated IgE responses to environmental, drug, or microbial antigens. Reexposure to even minute amounts of these antigens may trigger release of mast-cell products locally or systemically. The specific IgE-mast-cell complexes are so persistent that such a response to an antigen may occur long after the synthesis of IgE directed against that antigen has ceased. Individuals who exhibit such responses are said to be allergic to the inducing antigens. Such reactions often are called *atopic* or *anaphylactic.* The IgE antibodies previously were called *reaginic* antibodies, and antigens that induce these reactions were called *allergens.* The pathological manifestations of IgE-antigen interaction are due to mast-cell degranulation resulting in the release of histamine, heparin, slow-reacting substance A (SRS-A), a substance that constricts some smooth muscle cells over a prolonged interval, and a chemotactic factor for eosinophilic leukocytes. Pathological allergic reactions differ from other antibody reactions by their independence of complement, by their induction in response to minute doses of antigen, by their production of vascular and smooth muscle effects that appear in minutes, rather than hours, and by their susceptibility to prevention with antihistamines and to treatment with epinephrine. Epinephrine prevents mast-cell degranulation by raising cellular cAMP levels, and also antagonizes the action on smooth muscle of histamine and SRS-A. Allergic diseases may have systemic or local manifestations, depending on the route of entry of the antigen and the pattern of deposition of IgE and mast cells. Most local manifestations occur on epithelial surfaces, at the site of entry of the allergen. Allergic individuals characteristically give rapid responses in skin testing, have high serum IgE levels, and often have increased blood and tissue concentrations of eosinophilic leukocytes.

1.   *Systemic anaphylaxis* (anaphylactic shock) results from an IgE-basophil (blood mast cell) response to antigen in the circulation. The release of mast-cell mediators produces a biphasic response of vasoconstriction followed by peripheral vessel dilation. The result is a pooling of blood in the periphery and a concomitant drop in blood pressure (shock).

2.   *Food allergies* involve intestinal IgE-mast-cell responses to ingested antigens. These responses may affect the upper gastrointestinal tract, causing vomiting, or the lower gastrointestinal tract, causing cramps and diarrhea. If sufficient antigen is ingested, systemic anaphylaxis and skin reactions may occur.

3.   Skin reactions of the IgE-mast cell system may be acute or chronic. If acute, they may be a cause of *hives* (urticaria); if chronic, they may result in atopic dermatitis, a type of eczema. The basis for the latter condition is still unclear.

4.   Allergic reactions of the upper respiratory tract usually are grouped together and called hayfever (*allergic rhinitis*). Some patients affected by this condition develop large nasal polyps, which presumably result from chronic atopic reactions to nasal allergens.

5.   Reactions of the lower respiratory tract usually center in the bronchi and bronchioles, causing constriction and airway obstruction, and are a major cause of *asthma.* The acute effects probably are due to histamine release, and the long-term effects probably are due to SRS-A.

6.   Biting and stinging insects cause more damage by provoking allergic reactions than by direct action of their venom toxins. Individuals who are sensitized to these toxins may suffer fatal anaphylactic shock as the result of a bee sting.

B.   IgE-mediated diseases usually are treated by *desensitization,* the injection at intervals of just suballergic doses of the allergen. There are two likely explanations for the mechanism of desensitization. Treatment could induce an IgG response that competes with IgE for the allergen; or desensitization could induce specific T_S cells that suppress the synthesis of IgE directed against the allergen. Receptor blockade with *monovalent, nonmetabolizable* antigens may prove to be another approach to desensitization. This approach would prevent expression of an existing allergy by inactivating IgE-mast-cell complexes, and would prevent further production of IgE antibodies by blockading B_ε cells.

7-14   The predilection for some immunologic diseases is genetically linked to the MHC

A.   The finding that human leukocyte antigens (HLA) are important in tissue transplantation (Essential Concept 5–1) stimulated widespread investigation into the numbers and genetic relationships of these antigens. As previously explained, the major histocompatibility complex (MHC) which codes for these antigens was found to be highly polymorphic.

Table 7—2

Examples of associations between particular diseases and the MHC in humans

Disease	Linked MHC determinant (region)	Disease risk of persons who bear determinant (relative to disease risk in the population at large = 1)	Description of disease
Inflammatory diseases:			
Ankylosing spondylitis	W27 (HLA-B)	100–200	Inflammation of the spine, leading to stiffening of vertebral joints
Reiter's syndrome	W27 (HLA-B)	40	Inflammation of the spine, prostate, and parts of the eye (the uvea, which is the iris, the ciliary body, and the choroid)
Acute anterior uveitis	W27 (HLA-B)	30	Inflammation of the iris and ciliary body
Juvenile rheumatoid arthritis (Type II)	W27 (HLA-B)	10–12	A multisystem inflammatory disease of children characterized by joint disease, fever, and rapid onset
Psoriasis	A13 (HLA-B)	4–5	An acute, recurrent, localized inflammatory disease of the skin (usually scalp, elbows, knees), often associated with arthritis
Celiac disease	A8 (HLA-B)	9–10	A chronic inflammatory disease of the small intestine; probably a food allergy to gluten, a protein in grains
Multiple sclerosis	LD7a (HLA-D)	5	A progressive chronic inflammatory disease of brain and spinal cord that causes hardening (sclerosis) and loss of function in affected foci
Allergy:			
Ragweed hayfever	Many loci; direct linkage shown in family studies	difficult to calculate	An IgE-mediated allergic response to ragweed extracts
Endocrine diseases:			
Addison's disease	A8 (HLA-B)	4	A deficiency in production of adrenal gland cortical hormones
Diabetes mellitus (Juvenile)	A8, W15 (HLA-B) LD8a, LDW15a (HLA-D)	2–5	A deficiency of insulin production; pancreatic islet β cells usually absent or damaged
Graves' disease	LD8a (HLA-D)	10–12	A hyperactivity of the thyroid; patients often produce an IgG antibody that stimulates thyroid function (LATS: long-acting thyroid stimulator)
Malignant diseases:			
Acute lymphocytic leukemia	A2 (HLA-A)	1.2–1.4	A cancer of lymphocytes, usually in children, and usually of the T-lymphocyte series
Hodgkin's disease	A1 (HLA-A)	1.5–1.8	A cancer of lymph node cells; local inflammation is prominent, as well as selective deficiency in cellular immunity and T-cell functions

It was observed that certain MHC determinants occurred with high frequencies in association with certain diseases. Table 7–2 lists diseases that show significant associations with particular MHC determinants. Although this list is based on recent evidence and is incomplete, it suggests that molecules encoded by the MHC may play a role in certain diseases.

B.   It is not yet known which of the diseases in Table 7–2 are associated with immune response genes, human HLA-D determinants (the human equivalent of mouse Ia glycoprotein), and which with HLA-A, HLA-B, and HLA-C (the human equivalent of the mouse H-2D and H-2K glycoproteins). Knowledge of these specific associations undoubtedly will influence investigation into the etiology of the corresponding diseases.

   1.   Diseases associated with HLA-D and immune response genes could involve too little or too much of an immune response to a particular antigen. If such diseases are found, an understanding of their etiology may depend upon a resolution of the cellular and molecular basis of Ir gene action (Essential Concept 4–5).

   2.   Diseases associated with HLA-A, -B, and -C determinants could involve any of several phenomena. A particular MHC determinant could be the target of an autoimmune response, induced in one of the ways outlined in Essential Concept 7–9. T-cell-associated recognition of a particular MHC determinant could be unusual, resulting in an inappropriately high or low response to cells that bear associated antigens. MHC structures could serve as sites for attachment and entry of potentially pathogenic viruses. If the MHC is important for nonimmunologic cell interactions during development, then some MHC determinants might cause inappropriate development.

   Conceivably some of the extensive polymorphism of MHC determinants could be the result of their associations with diseases, which constitute a powerful selective force in evolution.

C.   Medical practice and research have given us a well-defined taxonomy of diseases, with detailed phenomenological descriptions of each disease. In contrast, most nonhuman animal diseases have received little or no study. Thus it is likely that the function and significance of the MHC genes will be elucidated at least partly from clues provided by investigation of human disease.

Selected Bibliography

Dixon, F. J., "Mechanisms of immunologic injury," in *Immunobiology* (ed. Good, R. A., and Fisher, D. W.), Ch. 22, Sinauer Associates, Inc., Stamford, Connecticut, 1971. An article on the biological aspects of antibody-mediated, complement-dependent immunological injury.

Fudenberg, H. H., Stites, D. P., Caldwell, J. L., and Wells, J. V., *Basic and Clinical Immunology*, Lange Medical Publications, Los Altos, Calif., 1978. Clinical immunology and immunopathology are rapidly becoming independent disciplines. This text covers these expanding fields in extensive clinical and histopathologic detail. It is useful as a well-written, current reference book, and is probably most valuable for students of clinical medicine and practicing physicians.

Hitzig, W. H., "Congenital immunodeficiency diseases: pathophysiology, clinical appearance and treatment," *Pathobiol. Annu.* **6,** 163 (1976). A recent review, focusing on clinical manifestations.

Louis, J. A., and Weigle, W. O., "A model of immunologic unresponsiveness and its relevance to autoimmunity," *Pathobiol. Annu.* **6,** 259 (1976). The latest in a series of perceptive articles by Weigle on the mechanisms involved in self-nonself discrimination.

Norman, P. S., "The clinical significance of IgE," *Hosp. Pract.* **8,** 41 (August 1975). A current view of the molecules, cells, and mediators responsible for allergy.

Exercises

7–1   Indicate whether each of the following statements is true or false. Explain the error in each statement you consider to be false.

F   (a)   Chronic granulomatous disease is a phagocytic cell dysfunction caused by defective membrane receptors for IgG and IgM Fc regions.

T   (b)   Recurrent pneumonia in patients with *cystic fibrosis* (a disease in which thickened mucous secretions prevent normal mucous flow) is a good example of failure of a general host defense mechanism.

T   (c)   The blood of children with Bruton's Disease (X-linked agammaglobulinemia) usually lacks mature B cells.

F   (d)   Antagonists of mast-cell degranulation can inhibit the development of kidney disease in systemic lupus erythematosis (SLE).

F   (e)   Contact sensitivity is a skin reaction that can be transferred passively with reaginic (IgE) antibody.

T (f) Lymphocytic choriomeningitis virus is nonlethal in thymus-deprived hosts.

T (g) The immunopathological injury formerly associated with rabies virus vaccination involved the activation of an autoimmune process.

F (h) Clinically, patients treated with antilymphocyte serum (ALS) would be expected to show a rapid decrease in circulating long-lived antibodies, for example, antibodies to polio virus.

F (i) Patients who lack the enzyme adenosine deaminase have a selective deficit in development of plasma cells (plasmacytopoiesis).

F (j) The predisposition for ankylosing spondylitis is genetically linked to the major blood-group antigen locus, ABO.

7–2 Supply the missing word or words in each of the following statements.

(a) The lack of an appropriate immune response to infection in the case of severe combined immunodeficiency is due to the failure in development of __T__ and __B__ cells.

(b) Rheumatoid arthritis is associated with serum antibodies, usually of the __IgM__ class, which react against __IgG Immunoglob.__

(c) Patients with hayfever have abnormal concentrations of __IgE__ antibodies, which, upon combination with their cognate antigen, activate __mast cells__.

(d) Linear deposition of antigen–antibody complexes on the glomerular basement membrane is detected by fluorescent anti-IgG antibody in __Goodpastures syndrome__

(e) As a pharmacologist, you wish to prepare a cytotoxic agent to be used as a preventative for people with bee-sting sensitivity. The purpose of your agent will be to eliminate __mast__ cells.

(f) __hereditary angioneurotic edema__ is a disease of complement regulation. The disease involves recurrent, local episodes of acute inflammation, which may be fatal when they affect the larynx.

(g) Skin lesions caused by poison oak involve an immune hypersensitivity of the __T cell__ system.

(h) Patients who develop progressive vaccinia viral infections following vaccination for smallpox most likely suffer from a disease that affects __T__ lymphocytes.

(i) C3 deficiency results in a decreased resistance to __bacterial__ infections.

(j) Systemic lupus erythematosis results in immunological injury to several organs because of the production of __immune complexes__.

Answers are given on page 157.

8 CANCER BIOLOGY AND IMMUNOLOGY

This chapter begins by describing the properties of cancer cells and of the agents that transform normal cells into malignant tumors. The subsequent sections deal with immune-related aspects of cancer: tumor-specific cell-surface changes that act as antigens to the host, the role of the immune system in immunosurveillance and elimination of cancers, the mechanisms by which cancers escape immunosurveillance, and the future of immunological approaches to the therapy, diagnosis, and prevention of cancer.

Essential Concepts

8-1 Cancer cells divide when they should not

A. Normal cell growth is regulated *in vivo* so that the proportion of proliferating cells in an organ increases or decreases to just balance the rates of cell loss, thereby maintaining constant organ size. Cancer cells do not respond to such regulation; consequently a higher proportion of their descendants continue to proliferate (Figure 8–1) and can give rise to large masses called tumors. A tumor (designated by the suffix *-oma*) is a swelling that may be due to cancer, inflammation, or infection. A tumor caused by cellular proliferation is called a neoplasm (new growth). Neoplasms that invade surrounding tissues and ultimately spread throughout the body are called *malignant neoplasms,* or *cancers.* Neoplasms that form noninvasive tumors, which do not spread to distant sites, are called *benign neoplasms.* Tumors that arise from epithelial cells are called *carcinomas* (Figure 8–2), and those that arise from stromal or mesenchymal cells are called *sarcomas* (Figure 8–3).

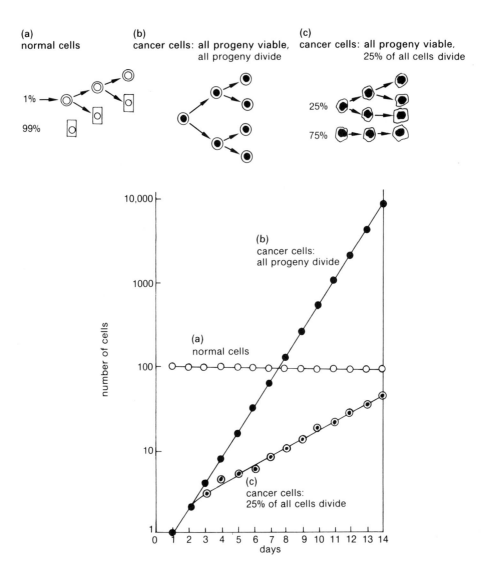

Figure 8–1 Growth kinetics of normal and neoplastic cells. Tissues composed of normal cells undergo a 1% loss per day, which is compensated by division of a small number of stem cells (a). If a normal stem cell becomes a cancer cell, it can proliferate by either a rapid completely exponential expansion (b) or a slower partially exponential expansion (c) to form a tumor.

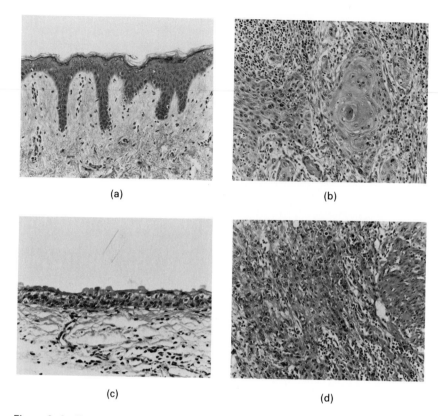

(a)

(b)

(c)

(d)

Figure 8–2 Examples of carcinomas and their normal counterparts. (a) A section of skin with normal epidermis showing orderly maturation from a row of basal cells to layers of thin, dead surface cells which form a protective layer. (b) Invasive skin carcinoma composed of cells with frequent mitoses. Disorderly maturation is exhibited by the whorls of cells in the center of a mass of tumor cells, rather than on the surface as seen in normal epidermis. (c) Normal lining cells of the bladder (transitional epithelium) consisting of lower layers of cuboidal-shaped cells and a single top layer of flattened cells. (d) Malignant transitional cell carcinoma arising in the lining of the bladder. The cells are invading the underlying tissue as cohesive but irregular masses. [Photographs courtesy of R. Rouse.]

8-2   Cancer cells invade other tissues

A.   The spread of cancer cells from the original transformed focus to distant organs is termed *metastasis*. The property of metastasis appears to be related to the nature of the original transformed focus, and is inherited by the progeny of the metastatic cells. The first stage of metastasis is the invasive extension of cancer cells into surrounding tissues. The second stage is the invasion of a vessel wall and the entry of cancer cells into either the lymphatic or the blood vascular system (Figure 8–4).

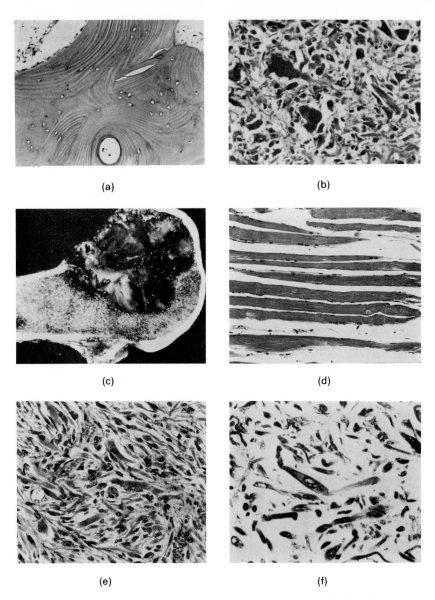

Figure 8–3 Examples of sarcomas and their normal counterparts. (a) Normal bone, consisting of regular layers of calcified matrix. Very few cells are present; they include individual bone cells (osteocytes) within spaces and a row of bone-forming cells (osteoblasts) on the surface. (b) The histologic appearance of a malignant osteosarcoma, showing increased cellularity, with numerous large, wild-looking cells. In some areas the cells are laying down irregular, uncalcified bone matrix (upper left corner). (c) A low-power view of an osteosarcoma, in a typical location, at the end of the femur. The malignant neoplasm can be seen invading the medullary cavity as well as eroding the cortex of the bone. Extensive bleeding and tissue death is common in these tumors. (d) Normal skeletal muscle with small, regular nuclei on the outer surfaces of the fibers. Cross striations are visible in most of the fibers. (e) The histologic appearance of a malignant rhabdomyosarcoma (sarcoma of rod-shaped [rhabdo] muscle [myo] cells), consisting of cells with centrally located, large, abnormally shaped nuclei. Some of the cells exhibit cross striations in their cytoplasm. (f) A higher-power view of a rhabdomyosarcoma, showing a cell with prominent cross striations. [Photographs courtesy of R. Rouse and P. Horne.]

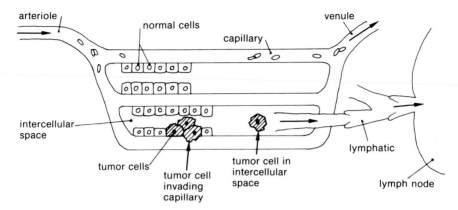

Figure 8-4 Diagrammatic view of the routes of tumor-cell invasion and the implications of these routes for the sites of distant metastases. Tumor cells that break off the original focus into the intercellular space enter afferent lymphatics and lodge in draining lymph nodes. Tumor cells that invade adjacent blood vessels enter the bloodstream and are distributed throughout the body.

1. Lymphatic vessels drain all intercellular fluid spaces in the body, conducting both particulate matter and plasma fluid into lymph nodes (Essential Concept 3-3). Cancer cells that break free from a tissue or invade a lymphatic vessel almost always become trapped in the meshwork of a draining lymph node. If these cancer cells proliferate, the result is abnormal enlargement of the lymph node (lymphadenopathy). Continued cancer cell proliferation may result in release of cancer cells into the efferent lymphatic vessel leading from the lymph node to the next lymph node up the chain. Eventually, cancer cells may enter a large collecting lymphatic such as the thoracic duct, which empties directly into the larger veins leading to the heart. Thus unchecked lymphatic metastases can lead to escape of cancer cells into the bloodstream.

2. Cancer cells also may invade blood vessels (Figures 8-4 and 8-5), and thereby enter the bloodstream directly. Cancer cells that enter the bloodstream and lodge in distant sites are called hematogenous (born from the blood) metastases.

8-3 The development of cancer cells may involve change or activation of the cellular genome

Carcinogenesis, the process by which cancers arise, is still poorly understood. The conversion of a normal cell to a cancer cell is called *transformation.* Because transformation is a property of the cancer cell and its clonal progeny, the process of transformation must involve

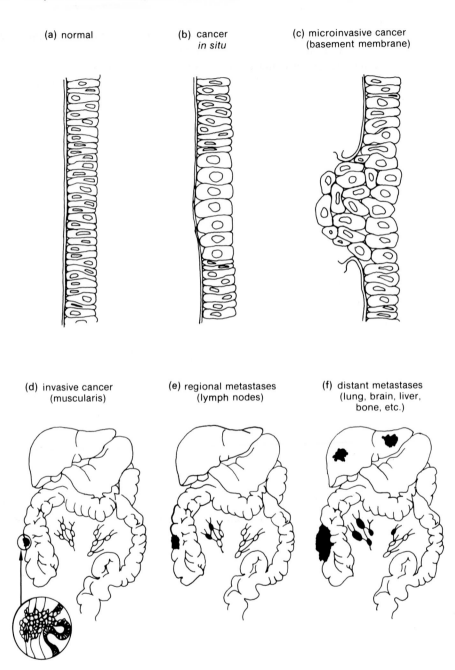

Figure 8–5 Successive stages in the development of a cancer of the colon (lower intestine). Going from left to right with time, an abnormal focus of cells invades the deeper muscular layer of the intestinal wall. spreads to local lymph nodes via the tissue lymphatics, and then to the liver following entry into blood vessels. ([Adapted from N. Berlin, *Hosp. Prac.* **10(1),** 83 (1975).]

the cell's genetic information. The two principal theories of carcinogenesis propose that transformation involves either *mutational* events, changing the genetic material, or *selective activation* of latent genes whose expression leads to the uncontrolled proliferation characteristic of cancer cells. In either case, the preclinical development of a cancer involves a *progression* of transformations, giving rise to successive subclones of increasing malignancy.

8-4   Some chemical and physical agents reproducibly cause cancer

A.   Epidemiological studies of cancer first suggested that substances in the environment could be responsible for carcinogenesis. Purification and fractionation of these substances sometimes led to loss of carcinogenic activity. Selective recombination of fractions, sometimes from separate sources (such as coal tar and cigarette smoke), restored activity. Such studies defined two classes of compounds active in chemical carcinogenesis: *carcinogens* and *promotors* (Table 8–1).

   1.   Carcinogens act rapidly on target cells. This event is necessary but not sufficient for the neoplastic transformation of the affected cell.

   2.   Promotors stimulate cell division of particular target cells. At least two cell-division cycles are required for malignant transformation of carcinogen-treated cells. Promotor action is reversible, and is not by itself carcinogenic. It must occur after carcinogen treatment to cause transformation.

B.   Although the mode of action of ultimate carcinogens in transformation is not yet established, there is increasing evidence that most if not all these compounds are potent mutagens. This generalization is the basis for the *Ames test,* a simple inexpensive screening procedure that can detect low levels of environmental carcinogens by their ability to increase the frequency of known mutational events in a bacterium such as *Salmonella.*

   The physical agents that cause cancer, such as ultraviolet and irradiation, also are highly mutagenic, acting directly on nucleic acids to cause genetic changes. Therefore, it seems likely that carcinogenic agents act on DNA to cause transformation, but whether their primary effect is through mutation or alteration of gene expression remains unresolved.

8-5   Genes that induce the malignant phenotype can be demonstrated in both DNA and RNA tumor viruses

A.   Certain DNA and RNA viruses, termed *oncogenic,* can transform the cells they infect and thereby induce tumor formation. There are several varieties of oncogenic DNA viruses, ranging from very simple

Table 8–1
Some common carcinogens and promotors

Class of compound	Carcinogens	Typical source	Promotors	Typical source
Polycyclic aromatic hydrocarbons	3,4-Benzpyrene (BP)	Coal tar; cigarette smoke; soot	Phorbolmyristate acetate (PMA)	Croton oil
	Methylcholanthrene (MC)	Coal tar; cigarette smoke; soot	Natural hormones	Ovary, adrenal, etc.
	Aflatoxin B_1	Aspergillus flavus (a fungus that grows on grains and peanuts)		
Aromatic amines	Dimethylaminobenzene (butter yellow; DAB)			
	2-Acetylaminofluorene (AAF)			
Food preservatives	Nitrates convert secondary amines to nitrosamines	Preserved meats such as frankfurters		
Azo dyes		Dye industry		
Irradiation	X ray	Military; nuclear reactors; medical diagnosis		
	Ultraviolet	Sun		
Other chemicals	Asbestos	Insulating material		
	Bis (2-chlorethyl) sulfide (mustard gas)	Military		
	Vinyl chloride	Plastics industry		
Drugs	Diethylstilbesterol	Medical therapy		

Table 8–2
Some DNA oncogenic viruses and their properties

Class	Virus	Genome size (molecular weight)	Host cell for productive infection	Host cell for *in vitro* malignant transformation
Papova	SV40 (Simian virus 40)	3×10^6	Monkey	Human, mouse, hamster
	Polyoma (poly = many, oma = tumors)	3×10^6	Mouse	Mouse, hamster, rat
	Papilloma (causes the benign skin tumors called warts)	5×10^6	?	Rabbit, human
Adenoviruses	Several types (e.g., adenovirus-12)	25×10^6	Human	Hamster, rat, human
Herpes	Herpes saimiri	100×10^6	?	Monkey
	Lucke carcinoma	100×10^6	?	Frog
	Marek's disease	100×10^6	?	Chicken
	Epstein-Barr virus (EBV)	100×10^6	Human (infectious mononucleosis)	Human? (Burkitt's lymphoma)

to very complex. A classification of these viruses and the neoplasms they induce is given in Table 8–2. The simplest viruses, SV40 and polyoma, have been analyzed most completely, and are therefore most useful for elucidating general principles. A small fraction of these cells undergo malignant transformation. The transformed cells retain one or a few viral genomes, integrated covalently into the host genome. It is not known whether any of the DNA oncogenic viruses (except papilloma virus) cause cancer in humans.

B.   Oncogenic RNA virus (*oncornavirus*) infections differ from DNA tumor virus infections in several respects. A unique set of enzymes coded for and carried by all oncornaviruses provides for the synthesis of a double-stranded circular DNA copy of the RNA genome called the *provirus*, which becomes inserted into the host cell genome (Figure 8–6) with concomitant transformation of the host cell. Oncornavirus-infected cells continually produce progeny virus by a budding process at the cell membrane. During budding the viral core is in the shape of an inverted C; hence these viruses are called C-type viruses (Figure 8–7). Like DNA oncogenic viruses, there are several varieties of oncornaviruses. A classification of these viruses and the neoplasms they produce is shown in Table 8–3.

The structural glycoproteins of the cell membrane budding site, which become the envelope glycoproteins of the virus, are coded by the viral genome. These molecules apparently organize into a cell membrane complex which largely, if not completely, excludes host cell membrane proteins. This budding site appears to be recognized

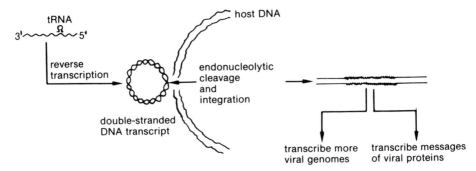

Figure 8–6   Events in the reverse transcription and integration of oncornavirus genes into host genomes. The enveloped virus penetrates into the target-cell cytoplasm. Using an enzyme called *reverse transcriptase,* which it codes for and carries with it, the virus begins the transcription of its RNA nucleotide sequence template into a complementary DNA nucleotide sequence. The reaction requires a primer, a host-cell transfer RNA (tRNA), which binds to a complementary sequence near the 5′ end of the viral RNA. A single-strand DNA is copied to the 5′ end of the viral RNA, and then synthesis continues, beginning at the 3′ end of the viral RNA. During this process the used viral RNA template is digested or removed, and a second-strand DNA copy is made using the reverse transcribed DNA as a template. The result is a double-stranded closed-circular proviral DNA copy of the viral RNA information. In cells susceptible to infection by this virus, the DNA provirus apparently integrates into a unique site in host chromosomal DNA, where it may act as a site of transcription of new viral RNA's and individual gene messages.

Table 8–3

A list of oncornaviruses and their effects

Name	Susceptible species	Type of tumor induced
Rapidly transforming viruses:		
Rous sarcoma virus	Chickens; other aves	Sarcomas
Moloney sarcoma virus	Rodents	Sarcomas
Friend focus-forming virus	Rodents	Erythro and myelomonocytic tumors
Abelson leukemia virus	Rodents	Hematopoietic tumors; B-cell tumors?
Simian sarcoma virus	Simians	Sarcomas
Slowly transforming viruses:		
Avian leukosis virus	Chickens	Lymphoid leukemia
Gross leukemia virus	Rodents	T-cell leukemias
Radiation leukemia virus	Rodents	T-cell leukemias
Friend lymphatic leukemia virus	Rodents	T-cell leukemias
Moloney leukemia virus	Rodents	T-cell leukemias
Feline leukemia virus	Cats; baboons?	Leukemias
Bovine leukemia virus	Cattle	Leukemias
Mouse mammary tumor virus	Rodents	Mammary carcinomas

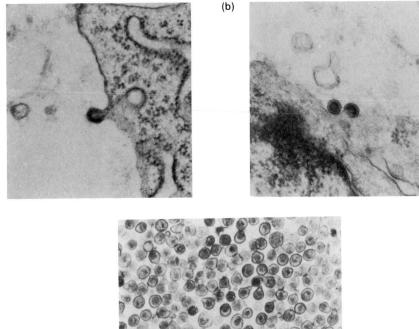

(a)   (b)

(c)

Figure 8–7 The budding of an oncornavirus. In (a) the virion bud is in the characteristic C-configuration, whereas in (b) one completed virion is adjacent to a nearly completed particle. In (c) a concentrate of these viruses is shown. [Photographs courtesy of O. Witte and D. Rice.]

specifically by cytoplasmic viral core assemblies that contain the virion RNA. Budding occurs by evagination of the core-membrane complex, ending with a separation and fusion of viral and cellular membranes (Figure 8–8). Oncornaviruses, like DNA tumor viruses, have not yet been conclusively demonstrated to cause cancer in humans.

8–6   Three kinds of methods currently are employed for treatment of cancer in humans

Two of the commonly used therapeutic approaches are localized, and one is systemic.

1. The primary method of localized cancer therapy is surgical removal of cancerous organs and tissues. This approach obviously requires a precise knowledge of the location and extent of the cancer, because only limited amounts of tissue can be excised.

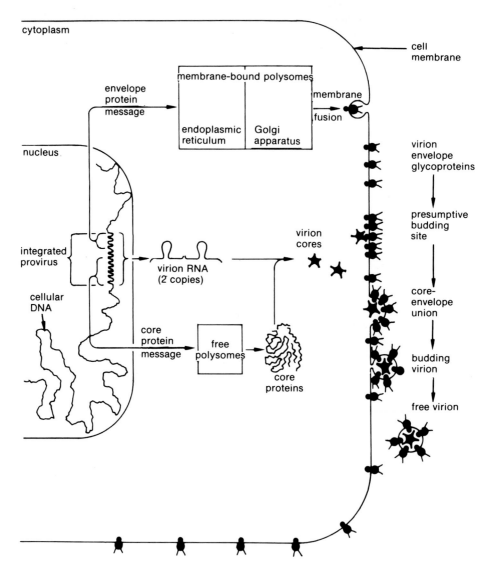

Figure 8–8 Cellular formation of oncornavirus budding sites. Virion mRNA's of two classes, core and envelope, are transcribed from integrated viral DNA copies. A core polyprotein is produced from core mRNA in the free polysome fraction, and is cleaved into several distinct proteins which combine with virion RNA to form the virion cores. Simultaneously, envelope mRNA is translated in polysomes bound to membranes of endoplasmic reticulum. This envelope precursor polyprotein is glycosylated, cleaved to its functional subunits, and inserted into the plasma membrane of the cell at presumptive budding sites. Core assemblies bind to the inner surface of presumptive budding sites and evaginate through them, with eventual separation of viral and cellular membranes.

2.   The second method of localized therapy is the application of ionizing radiation (radiotherapy) to the site of known primary and suspected metastatic sites. The radiation results in irreparable damage to cellular DNA; those cells that enter the next cell cycle are unable to complete mitosis and die (mitotic death). A few cell types, such as lymphocytes, die without mitosis within hours after absorbing a lethal dose of irradiation (interphase death). Radiotherapy also requires precise knowledge of tumor location and extent. This treatment is most useful against tumors of lymphoid origin with known metastatic patterns, such as Hodgkin's Disease, which now can be cured in up to 80% of all cases. Radiotherapy is also useful where an important structure must be cleared of cancer cells, but subsequently can function without extensive cell division. For example, radiotherapy for laryngeal carcinoma leaves the patient with intact, functioning vocal cords, whereas the surgical approach usually does not.

3.   The third method of cancer treatment is chemotherapy, the systemic administration of cytotoxic drugs. These drugs are designed to affect proliferating cells preferentially by interfering with pyrimidine and purine metabolism, DNA synthesis, or the process of mitosis (Figure 8-9). Because these drugs are accessible to all cells, malignant and normal, their major limitation is that they kill normal cells.

4.   With one or more of these therapeutic approaches, a number of cancers now can be cured that were incurable ten years ago. However, these cures may only be partially effected by the therapeutic treatment. Many oncologists believe that all cancer therapies act to reduce the tumor cell load to a size that host defense mechanisms can handle. In any case, curative cancer therapy must have as its goal the removal of all cancer cells, because a single cancer cell left unimpeded will multiply to kill the patient.

8-7   Most cancers are antigenic in their host of origin

A.   In 1908 the famous biologist Paul Ehrlich postulated that cancer cells arise frequently, and that they bear membrane changes that could be recognized as foreign antigens by the host. He further stated that the cellular immune response may in most cases be sufficient for cancer cell rejection. Fifty years later Lewis Thomas postulated that the development of cell-mediated immunity in evolution was driven by the need for *immunological surveillance* of newly arising neoplasms.

B.   Tumor antigenicity and host immunity to tumors was first demonstrated by a three-stage experiment (Figure 8-10). A carcinogen-induced

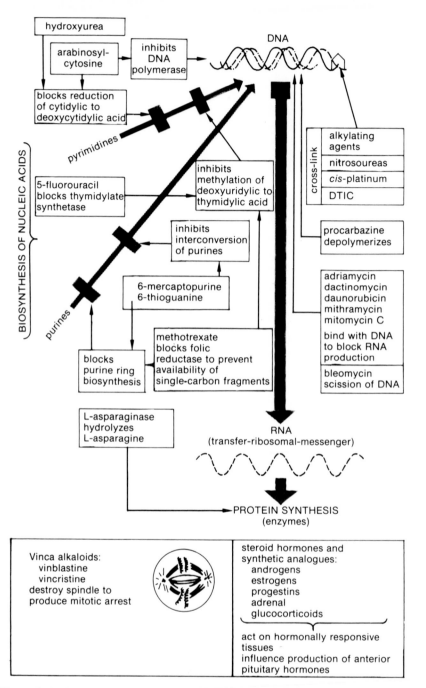

Figure 8–9 The actions of currently used anticancer chemotherapeutic agents. Three classes of agents are depicted: those that interfere with DNA synthesis or replication, those that affect the mitotic spindle and therefore arrest cells at metaphase, and those that act on tissues that require or are inhibited by steroid hormones. [Adapted from I. Krakoff, *Ca*—A Cancer Journal for Clinicians **27(3)**, 130 (1977).]

cancer was excised completely from its original host, and then varying numbers of tumor cells were transplanted to syngeneic hosts. The number of transplanted cells that reproducibly induced tumors in the recipient hosts was determined. Retransplantation of this number of tumor cells from the secondary hosts to the original host usually resulted in no tumor growth. This phenomenon was *specific* for the original tumor. Adoptive transfer of lymphocytes from the original host to genetically identical naive hosts conferred specific resistance to the original tumor. This transfer of immunity required the transfer of live lymphocytes, subsequently identified as T lymphocytes.

With the advent of sensitive techniques, such as immunofluorescence and radioimmunoassay, for assaying antibodies specific to tumor antigens, it was demonstrated that tumor-bearing hosts had both a cell-mediated and a humoral immune response to their own tumor antigens. The resulting humoral antibodies were used in cross-absorption studies to compare large numbers of tumors and normal cells. Thus it was possible to identify tumors with *cross-reacting antigens,* tumors with *tumor-unique antigens,* and tumors with antigens common to a subset of normal cells (*differentiation antigens*).

C. In theory, apparent tumor-specific antigens could be new determinants or simply very rare normal determinants. Most tumors are populated predominantly by a single clone of cells, all of which share the cell-membrane properties of the original transformed cell. Some of the surface determinants of each normal cell may be unique, or shared by only a few other cells. If so, the concentration of these unique determinants will be far too low to trigger either an immunogenic or tolerogenic response. However, if such a cell gives rise to a transformed clone of identical cells, its surface molecules may provoke an immune response even if no new determinants are present. Thus a carcinogen-induced transformation may produce a change in the cell surface, or simply may select for expansion of a rare subset of preexisting cells bearing unique cell-surface determinants (Figure 8–11).

D. In experimental situations, four classes of tumor antigens are found. The first class is called oncofetal antigens. These antigens are found on the surfaces of cancer cells, but also are expressed during a specific phase of embryonic differentiation.

1. An important example is the carcinoembryonic antigens of the colon (CEA). This set of antigens is found on the surfaces of all tumor cells derived from the gastrointestinal tract or derivatives of the fetal gastrointestinal tract, such as pancreas, liver, and gall bladder. These antigens, which appear to be glycoproteins, have been demonstrated to be present on only a small subset of normal adult cells, so that the total body concentration of CEA normally is extremely small.

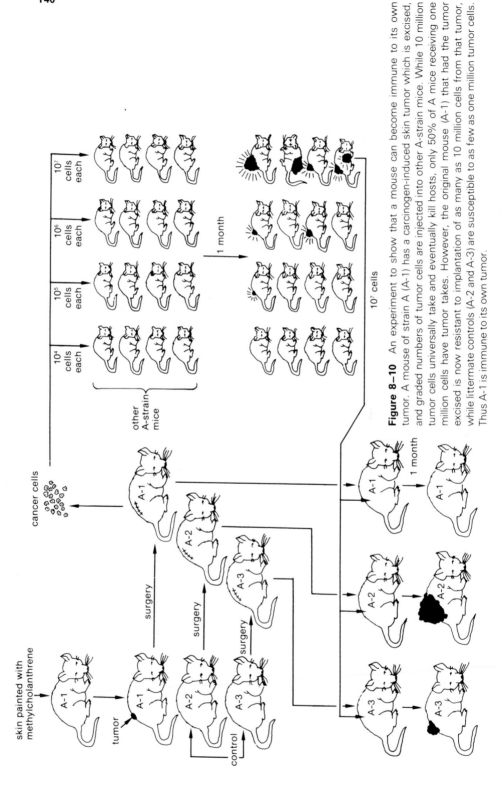

Figure 8–10 An experiment to show that a mouse can become immune to its own tumor. A mouse of strain A (A-1) has a carcinogen-induced skin tumor which is excised, and graded numbers of tumor cells are injected into other A-strain mice. While 10 million tumor cells universally take and eventually kill hosts, only 50% of A mice receiving one million cells have tumor takes. However, the original mouse (A-1) that had the tumor excised is now resistant to implantation of as many as 10 million cells from that tumor, while littermate controls (A-2 and A-3) are susceptible to as few as one million tumor cells. Thus A-1 is immune to its own tumor.

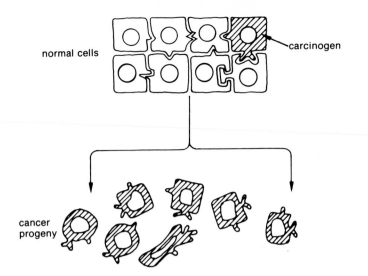

normal cells

carcinogen

cancer progeny

Figure 8–11 A clonal selection hypothesis to describe carcinogen-induced tumor-specific antigens. Several distinct cell types in a tissue adhere to each other by cell-specific surface properties. The carcinogen selectively transforms one of these types. The clonal progeny resulting from this transformation bear the same cell-specific determinants, but these cancer cells show a wide variety of morphological characteristics (pleomorphism). Because these malignant progeny no longer have complementary cells to adhere to, they tend to grow away from the original focus.

2. Another important example is alpha-fetoprotein (αFP), normally secreted by yolk sac and fetal liver epithelial cells, and also produced by malignant yolk sac and liver cells. Although αFP is a secreted product, anti-αFP immune responses restrict growth of these neoplasms. Careful analysis has revealed that αFP is not solely a tumor antigen in adults, but is normally expressed by the proliferating fraction of liver cells.

E. The second class of tumor-specific antigens is those induced by chemical carcinogens. Each carcinogen-induced tumor expresses unique cell-surface antigens. When a single mouse is skin-painted with the carcinogen methylcholanthrene at several different sites, each of the resulting carcinomas will express cell-surface antigens that are identical on all cells within the tumor but different from the antigens expressed by the other methylcholanthrene-induced tumors. Individual tumor-specific antigens are also found on tumors induced by any other chemical carcinogen.

There is also an important clinical aspect of the finding that carcinogens induce unique tumor-specific antigens. If each new carcinogen-induced tumor bears only unique tumor-specific determinants, then it will be difficult if not impossible to prepare in advance a stockpile of specific immunologic reagents for tumor detection or treatment.

F. The third class of tumor-associated antigens comprises those induced by oncogenic DNA viruses. Each of these viruses induces unique nuclear and cell-surface antigens in cells that it transforms. For a particular virus these antigens are always the same, regardless of differences in the tissue, the animal, or even the species in which the transformation occurs. The three major candidates for human DNA virus-induced tumors, Burkitt's lymphoma, nasopharyngeal carcinoma, and cancer of the cervix (the virus candidates are various herpes viruses), do express tumor-associated cell-surface antigens and the antigens are the same from one tumor to the next.

G.   The fourth class of tumor-associated antigens is those induced by oncornavirus transformation. Like the DNA tumor viruses, each RNA tumor virus induces specific antigens that are the same, regardless of differences in the host cell. However, unlike the DNA viruses, most, if not all, oncornavirus-specific tumor antigens are viral protein antigens. Some of these proteins represent precursors of virus budding sites on the transformed cell membrane (Figure 8-8). These antigens may have *group-specific* determinants in common with all viruses of a certain group, for example mouse leukemia viruses, *type-specific* determinants shared by only a few closely related viruses, for example Gross and Radiation leukemia viruses, and unique virus-specific determinants. These determinants may be present on various virion polypeptides; at least one cell-surface antigen is an internal virion protein.

Most of the leukemogenic oncornaviruses induce neoplasms that express normal differentiation antigens as well. In the mouse, one differentiation antigen, TL, may be anomalously expressed by thymic lymphomas from a mouse strain that normally does not express TL antigens on its thymocytes. Thus the control of TL expression somehow can be interfered with by oncornavirus-induced transformation.

8-8   Cancer cells are attacked by the cellular immune system

A.   The first experiment clearly to define the role of antibodies and cells in the immune response to cancers was carried out in the late 1940's. Cancer cells were placed into a cell-impermeable chamber with pores 0.2 μ in diameter that allowed molecules, but not cells, to enter and exit. When the chambers were placed into hosts immune to the cancer cells, the cells survived and multiplied, although high concentrations of cancer-specific antibodies diffused into the chamber and bound to the cells. However, when the experiment was repeated with a chamber that contained pores large enough for cells to enter, the cancer cells were destroyed, and host lymphoid cells could be found infiltrating the tumor mass. These experiments provided the first evidence that most tumors are not susceptible to attack by antibodies alone or by antibodies plus complement, but that they are susceptible to attack by killer cells. Three kinds of killer cells may be involved in cell-mediated immunity to tumors: T_c cells, natural killer (NK) cells, and the cells responsible for antibody-dependent cell-mediated cytotoxicity (ADCC). In most cancers, the T_c response is dominant (see Essential Concept 4–6). However, leukemias are quite sensitive to natural killer cells, to antibody and complement, and to antibody-dependent cell-mediated cytotoxicity. In general, cancers of the hematolymphoid system are sensitive to both humoral and cellular immunity, whereas all other cancers are susceptible to cellular immunity only.

If the T-cell immune system is important for elimination of newly arising tumors, then animals and humans deficient in this system should be highly susceptible to induced tumors and also should have a high incidence of spontaneous tumors.

1. Animals deprived of their thymus early in life are indeed extremely susceptible to various oncogenic viruses. For example, when neonatally thymectomized mice are exposed to Moloney sarcoma virus or polyoma virus, the animals suffer a high incidence of tumors that grow more rapidly than the tumors induced at low incidence in nonthymectomized littermate controls. Furthermore, the tumors from thymectomized animals are more highly antigenic on a per cell basis than the tumors in nonthymectomized littermates. These results, and those described in the preceding section, fulfill a postulate of the immunosurveillance hypothesis, that is, that the immune system responds to the antigens of endogenous neoplasms.

2. Another postulate of the hypothesis, that the cellular immune system has evolved to protect against a high rate of spontaneously arising neoplasms, is more controversial. As improvements in animal husbandry have allowed congenitally athymic animals to survive longer, it has been found that they do not have a high incidence of death from cancer. Further experiments are needed to determine whether these animals have a thymus-independent immune response that is sufficient for immunosurveillance, whether there is a nonimmune surveillance mechanism for removal of antigenic or newly arising tumor cells, or whether the assumption that tumors frequently arise simply is not true.

3. Immunologically deficient humans suffer a strikingly high incidence of cancer. For example, nearly 10% of children with congenital immunological deficiency disease develop cancer. However, these cancers are principally derived from cells of the lymphoid system, and it is not certain whether the high rate of neoplasia is due to lack of immunosurveillance, or to pathological consequences of the lymphoid system imbalance.

4. The best documented examples of increased tumor incidence in immunosuppressed hosts come from patients treated with immunosuppressive drugs for allogeneic kidney transplants. These

patients have an eighty-fold increased risk of developing cancer; about 60% of their cancers are of epithelial origin and about 40% of lymphoid origin. Again, it is unclear whether these cancers reflect the patient's immunodeficient state, or result from a pathological lymphoid disorder. The results are further complicated by the observation that the frequencies of the various epithelial neoplasms that develop in these patients do not correspond to the frequencies found in other groups of patients matched for age, sex, and geographical location. For example, immunosuppression causes little increase in the incidence of breast cancer or lung cancer, whereas it causes large increases in the incidence of other epithelial neoplasms.

In summary, there is circumstantial evidence to support the immunosurveillance hypothesis, but the theory has not been conclusively tested. Still lacking is knowledge of all the immune mechanisms that could be involved, and proof that cancers arise spontaneously at a high frequency.

8-9   Some cancer cells escape immunological surveillance

A.   Whatever the general validity of the immunosurveillance hypothesis, by the time a tumor is diagnosed most cancer patients demonstrate both cellular and humoral immunity directed specifically at cell-surface antigens of the tumor cells. How then do these tumor cells survive in what should be a hostile environment? Tumor growth under these conditions has been termed immunologic escape. Several different mechanisms of immunologic escape have been found in research on experimental tumors; these studies form the basis for our current understanding of human tumor immunology.

    1. *Immunological tolerance:* Animals injected very early with tumors or high concentrations of tumor-associated antigens before the development of full immunological competence maintain a specific unresponsiveness to these tumors if they are transplanted into the animals later in life. This phenomenon appears to be identical to that of immunological tolerance described in Essential Concept 4–9.

    2. *Immunoselection:* Rare variant cells that have lost the original surface antigens occur in large tumor cell populations. In the face of an immune response against the antigenic tumor cells, the variants selectively grow to dominate the tumor. These cells may bear a different set of antigens and may in turn induce their own specific immune response. The immune response does not induce antigenic change; it merely selects for cells that have undergone antigenic change independently.

3. *Antigenic modulation:* This interesting phenomenon provides an example of how understanding the basic biology of microorganisms leads to an important clinical insight. In the 1940's Beale and Sonneborn observed that treatment of paramecia with antibodies specific for their ciliary antigens leads to cessation of movement. However, if the paramecia are metabolically active, they soon begin to swim again, even in the continued presence of antibody. Further examination reveals that they have lost the antigens formerly present on their cilia and are expressing a new set of antigens. In the presence of antibody to the new antigens, modulation may occur again, with either reexpression of the first antigens or expression of another new set of antigens. These ciliary antigens all are determined by nuclear genes of the paramecium.

Similar antigenic modulation has been demonstrated in two systems of mouse leukemic cells. Thymic leukemias induced in some mouse strains by thymotropic murine leukemia viruses express TL antigens. Transfer of these thymic leukemia cells to hosts immune to TL antigens does not stop progressive growth of the tumor. Analysis of the leukemia cells growing in these recipient hosts reveals no cell-surface TL antigens. In tissue culture as well, when anti-TL antibody is added to TL-positive leukemia cells they also lose the TL antigens, and within a few hours 100% of the cells are TL-negative. In the absence of anti-TL antibodies, the TL antigens usually reappear, indicating that both the controlling genes and the structural genes for the TL antigens remain intact in the modulating cells and in their descendants.

Immunoglobulin molecules on the surfaces of B cells and B-cell leukemias also are subject to antigenic modulation. In this case, it has been demonstrated directly that some of the original antigenic molecules are swept off the cell surface while others are removed from the cell surface by endocytosis.

4. *Immunostimulation:* In the 1950's it was first suggested that some aspect of the immune response against a tumor may actually trigger cancer cells into more rapid or extensive proliferation. Recently it has been demonstrated in a few tumor systems that a weak immune response may indeed promote increased outgrowth of antigenic tumor cells. The mechanism of this stimulation is not known.

5. *Immunosuppression:* There are at least two ways in which immunosuppression can occur in a cancer patient. The most common is iatrogenic immunosuppression, that is, immunosuppression caused by agents used to treat the cancer. Most anticancer agents, including ionizing radiation, and cytotoxic drugs, have as side effects the destruction of lymphocytes and other cells important in the generation and maintenance of immune responses.

In some cancers the tumors themselves seem to release immunosuppressive factors. The most striking example of this phenomenon is Hodgkin's disease, in which a small tumor in a single lymph node releases or induces the release of immunosuppressive factors that have a powerful effect on the entire cell-mediated immune system. Patients with Hodgkin's disease have a poor delayed hypersensitivity response and are abnormally sensitive to intracellular parasitic infections such as tuberculosis and Herpes virus infections.

6. *Immunological enhancement:* In some cases animals preimmunized with allogeneic grafts of disrupted cells from a certain tumor and subsequently challenged with the same tumor will support its growth and eventually die. Nonimmunized animals challenged with the same tumor will allow it only brief growth and then reject it. Several experiments suggest a diversity of mechanisms to explain this paradoxical finding.

Immunological enhancement of tumor allograft growth may be accomplished by passive transfer of serum from an immunized host to a syngeneic nonimmune host, even if antiserum injection is delayed until as late as seven days after tumor implantation. This result suggests that enhancement is due to blockade of the effector mechanisms that normally promote tumor rejection

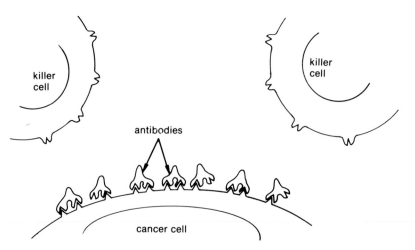

Figure 8–12 Blockade of effector (killer) cell function by competing antibodies directed against the same target-cell antigens that the killer cells recognize.

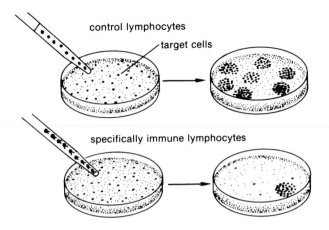

control lymphocytes

target cells

specifically immune lymphocytes

Figure 8–13 The colony inhibition test is predicated upon killing or growth inhibition of tumor cells by specifically immune lymphocytes. By comparing the number of colonies formed when immune lymphocytes are used with the number when control lymphocytes are used, the percentage of tumor cells killed or inhibited by the immune lymphocytes can be derived. [Adapted from K. E. and I. Hellström, "Immunologic defenses against cancer," in *Immunobiology*, R. A. Good and D. W. Fisher (Eds.), Sinauer Associates, Stamford, Conn., 1971, Chapter 21.]

(Figure 8–12). However, immunological enhancement also is observed if tumor cells precoated with enhancing antibodies are injected, suggesting that enhancement can operate by altering the initial sensitization mechanism. Experiments with an *in vitro* model system support the existence of serum blocking factors that interfere with effector-cell mechanisms. Growth of tumor cells in tissue culture normally is inhibited by lymphocytes from the tumor-bearing host (Figure 8–13). This lymphocyte effect can be blocked by addition of serum from the tumor-bearing host (Figure 8–14) but not by serum from hosts with another tumor type. This result could be due to blockade of tumor target-cell antigenic determinants by anti-tumor antibodies, which would prevent attack by immune lymphocytes. If so, these experiments appear to indicate a basic antagonism between humoral and cell-mediated immunity to tumors. Alternatively, the serum-blocking factors could be solubilized tumor-cell antigens, which either alone or complexed with anti-tumor antibodies inhibit immune lymphocytes by blockade or elimination reactions (Figure 8–15).

In some cases of immunological tolerance as well as immunological enhancement, the dominant influence in specific inhibition of the immune response appears to be suppression, that is, suppressor T cells or products of suppressor T cells. Thus it is possible that specific suppression also plays some role in the enhancement of tumor growth by inhibition of immune responses (Figure 8–16).

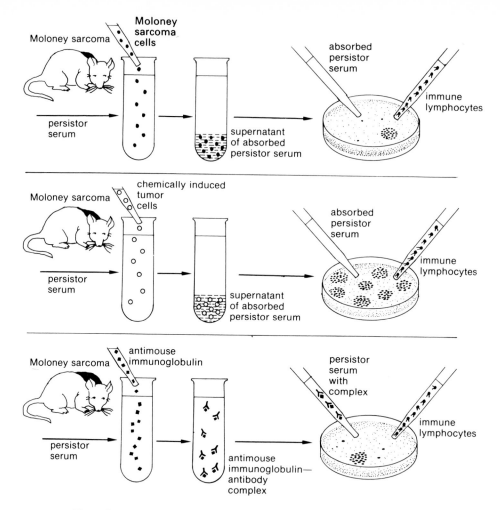

Figure 8–14 Two types of experiments provide evidence that the serum factors protecting persistent tumors contain specific antibodies. When serum from an animal with a Moloney sarcoma (persistor serum) is absorbed with Moloney sarcoma cells, the serum loses its ability to protect tumor cells (top). When cells from a different type of tumor (chemically induced) are used, the protective effect of the serum is unchanged (middle). The protective effect is also lost when added goat anti-mouse immunoglobulin complexes with serum antibody. [Adapted from K. E. and I. Hellström; see legend for Figure 8–13.]

8-10 Immunological approaches can contribute to the therapy, diagnosis, and prevention of cancer

A.   Given the complexity of immune responses in patients with clinically detectable tumors, what are the prospects for development of cancer immunotherapy? It is clear that humans usually have both a humoral and a cell-mediated immune response to their own tumor antigens, but that for some reason this response is not always effective.

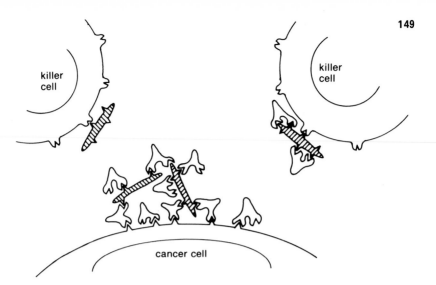

Figure 8–15 Two models of blocking-factor action. Antigen (shaded) or antigen–antibody complexes form lattices which may obscure target-cell antigenic determinants and/or killer-cell receptors.

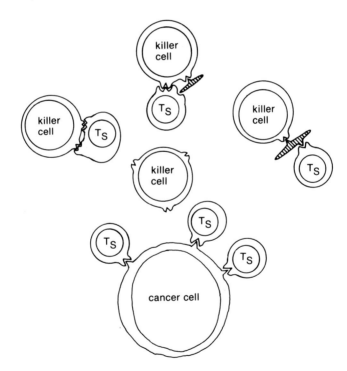

Figure 8–16 How suppressor T cells may block tumor immunity. T_s cells may affect T_c cells by having receptor specificity for T_c-cell idiotype, or for the combination of antigen with T_c idiotype, or for antigen alone. Alternatively, T_s cells may suppress by direct action on the tumor target cell, and thus have receptor specificity for tumor antigens.

1. Cell-mediated immunity provides the best defense against most cancers. However, attempts to increase the number of killer T cells and antibody-dependent killer cells in a patient may result in expansion of inhibitory cell clones as well. Moreover, because the dimensions of the blocking-factor problem are not yet understood, it is not clear that increased clones of killer cells could compete with the blocking system.

2. Adoptive transfer of immunity to human cancer antigens from one patient to the next by transfer of live lymphocytes could be exceedingly dangerous because of the probable graft-versus-host response to the recipient's transplantation antigens. Such a response affects several of the body's important organ systems, and is often fatal. Until it is possible to separate lymphocytes specific for normal cell targets from those specific for tumor cells this approach to immunotherapy will not be possible.

3. An approach currently being tested is called adjuvant immunotherapy. In this method the tumor is inoculated with BCG, an attenuated mycobacterium that is related to the tubercle bacillus and is an intracellular parasite of macrophages. The resulting immune response leads not only to the destruction of intracellular forms of BCG, but also to a massive increase in the number and activity of the phagocytic cells. BCG in combination with most immunogens heightens the immune response. In mice it slightly but significantly increases the immune response to tumors. BCG may act either as an immunological adjuvant by increasing the immunogenicity of the antigens it is mixed with, or by increasing the activity of the macrophage system. This increased activity could be nonspecific, or it could involve an increase in either natural killer cells or in the cells responsible for antibody-dependent cell-mediated immunity. Thus far the effect of BCG on human tumors seems limited to those accessible to injection or infection with BCG; distant metastases and internal tumors usually are unaffected. BCG is potentially dangerous because increasing the immunogenicity of tumor cell antigens could increase the levels of blocking factors or suppressor cells as well as the cell-mediated immune response against a tumor.

4. Antibody therapy of tumors also is impractical at this time. Injections of tumor-specific antibody into tumor-bearing hosts would be helpful only for leukemias, in which the cells are sensitive to antibody-triggered immunological destruction rather than to immunological enhancement, which otherwise is the most likely consequence of passive antibody transfer. Triggering antibody-dependent cell-mediated immunity would be another hypothetical

approach, but this possibility will be impractical until more is known about the requirements for effective antibody in the triggering process.

In summary, the current prospects for development of an effective cancer immunotherapy are not promising.

B.   By contrast, immunodiagnosis of cancer is likely to be an important addition to the clinician's armamentarium. Many tumors release specific cell-surface antigens into the bloodstream, and these antigens can be detected by radioimmunoassay (see Chapter 5). There are three important limitations to this type of assay: first, antigen must be available in highly purified form so that the radioimmunoassay will be specific; second, the determinants must retain antigenicity when radiolabeled with iodine; and third, the antigen must be free to enter the circulation in tumor-bearing hosts.

Immunoassay also can be used to measure levels of serum antibody to a specific tumor antigen. Assays that detect antibody action on whole tumor cells *in vitro* may be used, so that it is unnecessary that purified antigen be available or that the tumor release antigen into the circulation. It is necessary only that antibody responses be related in some way to the presence or absence of tumor antigens in the host.

C.   Immunological techniques also could be useful in cancer prevention. If it ever becomes possible to identify infectious agents, such as oncornaviruses that induce tumors bearing virus-specific antigens, then the possibility of vaccination with attenuated forms of these agents could be considered. However, as pointed out in Essential Concept 8–9, induction of an immune response to a tumor-associated antigen may result in immunological enhancement rather than in protective immunity. Extensive animal testing would be required to determine the potential benefits and risks of such an approach before it could be applied to humans. Whereas immunodiagnosis and immunotherapy would be applied to patients with poor prognoses, vaccination would be carried out on a healthy population. Large-scale vaccination could not be justified unless the risk of inducing disease was proven to be virtually nonexistent.

Selected Bibliography

Cairns, J., "The cancer problem," *Sci. Am.* **233**, 64 (1975) A general review of cancer biology, with emphasis on possible environmental causes of cancer.

Koprowski, H. (Ed.), *Neoplastic Transformation: Mechanisms and Consequences,* Pergamon Press, Berlin, 1977. A recent comprehensive review aimed at the nonexpert.

Nicolson, G. L., and Poste, G., "The cancer cell: dynamic aspects and modifications in cell-surface organization," *N. Engl. J. Med.* **295,** 197 (1976). A current review of cell-membrane changes associated with specific properties of cancer cells.

Heidelberger, C., "Chemical carcinogenesis," *Annu. Rev. Biochem.* **44,** 79 (1975). A comprehensive survey of the field, including consideration of carcinogens (and their metabolic activation) *in vivo* and *in vitro,* and discussion of their possible modes of action.

Rubin, H., "Carcinogenicity tests," *Science* **191,** 241 (1976).

Ames, B. N., "Reply," *Science* **191,** 241 (1976). Are carcinogens mutagens, and if so, does their mutagenicity explain their mode of action in malignant transformation? Two distinguished scientists from the University of California, Berkeley, debate the issue.

Dulbecco, R., "From the molecular biology of oncogenic DNA viruses to cancer," *Science* **192,** 437 (1976). A Nobel Prize lecture for 1975.

Baltimore, D., "Viruses, polymerases, and cancer," *Science* **192,** 632 (1976). A Nobel Prize lecture for 1975.

Temin, H. M., "The DNA provirus hypothesis," *Science* **192,** 1075 (1976). A Nobel Prize lecture for 1975.

Burnet, F. M., "The concept of immunological surveillance, *Prog. Exp. Tumor Res.* **13,** 1 (1970). A restatement of the Ehrlich hypothesis, with a more elaborate discussion of the possibility that immunosurveillance is the driving force for the T-cell immunity system.

Klein, G., "Tumor antigens," *Annu. Rev. Microbiol.* **20,** 223 (1966). Antigens induced by oncogenic viruses are common from tumor to tumor induced by a particular virus.

Klein, G., "Immunological surveillance against neoplasia," *Harvey Lecture Series* **69,** 71 (1975).

Exercises

8–1   Indicate whether each of the following statements is true or false. Explain the error in each statement you consider to be false.

~~F~~   (a)   Cancer cells generally divide more rapidly than normal cells.

~~F~~   (b)   Tumor-associated antigens that are expressed earlier in development as fetal membrane components cannot induce an immune response in the adult animal because of the lack of immunologic responsiveness to self-components (tolerance).

~~F~~   (c)   The spread of cancer viruses from one organ to another is called metastasis.

~~T~~   (d)   Each chemically induced tumor appears to have a unique tumor-associated antigen.

~~T~~   (e)   The lymphocytes from a patient dying of malignant melanoma usually can destroy his own tumor cells *in vitro*.

~~T~~   (f)   The lymphocytes from one patient with malignant melanoma usually can destroy *in vitro* the tumor cells from a second patient with this same disease.

8–2   Supply the missing word or words in each of the following statements.

(a)   Immunodiagnosis is based on the supposition that *tumor-assoc Ag* _____ _____ for distinct tumors are different.

(b)   Most anticancer drugs *suppress* the immune system.

(c)   DNA copies are made of the RNA virus genome by *reverse transcriptase* _____.

(d)   The rapid loss of most (if not all) copies of a cell-surface tumor antigen upon contact with specific antibody is called *Ag modulation* _____.

(e)   The cellular immune system may have evolved as a *surveillance* system for cancer.

(f)   Tumor-associated antigens that result in immune rejection usually are located in the cancer cell *plasma membrane*.

(g)   *Blocking factors* appear to be comprised of humoral antibodies and tumor-associated antigens.

Answers are given on pages 157–158.

Answers to Exercises

Chapter 1

1-1 (a) True
      (b) True
      (c) True
      (d) False. A hapten cannot stimulate antibody production by itself, but it can combine with specific antibody.
      (e) True
      (f) False. B cells, but not T cells, secrete antibody molecules.
      (g) False. The Fc region is the C-terminal half of the heavy chains.
      (h) True

1-2 (a) carrier   (e) heavy
      (b) Plasma cells   (f) vertebrates
      (c) cellular   (g) cognate
      (d) Humoral   (h) IgA, IgD, IgE, IgG, and IgM

Chapter 2

2-1 (a) False. The hinge region joins the N- and C-terminal halves of the heavy chain.
      (b) False. The light chains of a single antibody molecule always are identical, as are the heavy chains.
      (c) False. The V_L and V_H regions are approximately the same size.
      (d) True
      (e) False. Both chains contribute to the active site.
      (f) False. The C_H regions distinguish the classes and subclasses of antibodies.
      (g) False. The immune response to a single antigen usually consists of a heterogeneous array of different antibody molecules.
      (h) False. Identical myeloma proteins from different humans never have been observed.
      (i) True

2–2 (a) variable
     (b) somatic
     (c) Myeloma proteins
     (d) domains
     (e) hypervariable
     (f) effector; antigen-binding
     (g) lambda and kappa

Chapter 3

3–1 (a) True
     (b) False. B cells that enter the spleen home to follicles on the outside of the sheath.
     (c) True
     (d) True
     (e) False. T cells mature in the thymus; B cells probably mature in the bone marrow.
     (f) True
     (g) True
     (h) False. The primary follicles of lymph nodes are B-cell domains.

3–2 (a) antigen; antigen
     (b) macrophages; dendritic reticular cells
     (c) Cytotoxic; killer
     (d) Tolerance
     (e) Virgin
     (f) white pulp
     (g) afferent
     (h) dendritic reticular cells; macrophages
     (i) B
     (j) bursa of Fabricius
     (k) immunocompetent

Chapter 4

4–1 (a) False. IgG is the major class of antibody synthesized in a secondary response.
     (b) False. Genes that code for anti-self antibodies are inherited. Tolerance probably results from the elimination or paralysis of lymphocyte clones that produce anti-self antibodies.
     (c) False. Macrophages do not belong to the lymphocyte lineage and never differentiate into T cells.
     (d) False. C3 also can be activated by the alternate (properdin) pathway.
     (e) True
     (f) False. Macrophages also are required for a B-cell immune response.

(g) False.   The genes that code for antibody combining-site specificities (variable-region genes) are linked to allotypic markers, which
represent antibody constant-region genes. Ir genes are linked to the
major histocompatibility complex.

(h) True

4–2 (a) secondary
(b) Blast transformation
(c) T cells, B cells, and macrophages
(d) IgM
(e) immune response (Ir)
(f) receptor blockade
(g) IgE
(h) IgG

Chapter 5

5–1 (a) True
(b) False.   The point of maximum precipitation usually occurs at a
slight weight excess of antigen.
(c) True
(d) True
(e) False. A heterologous antiserum is raised in a different species
than the one that provided the test antibody.
(f) True
(g) True

5–2 (a) Immunoelectrophoresis
(b) β and γ
(c) Farr
(d) equilibrium dialysis
(e) A and B; A, B, AB, and O
(f) fluorescent, radioactive, enzymatic, or electron-opaque

Chapter 6

6–1 (a) False.   Transplants between identical twins are termed syngeneic
grafts. Because there is no mismatch in transplantation antigens, no
immunosuppression is required.
(b) True
(c) False.   Skin transplants are usually rejected by the cell mediated
immune system, whereas transfusion reactions involve an antibody-
mediated elimination of blood cells.

(d) False. In the first trimester the fetus is immunodeficient, and therefore cannot cause an immunological rejection of maternal lymphocytes. It is likely that these maternal lymphocytes would cause a fatal multisystem graft-versus-host reaction against the fetus.
(e) True

6–2 (a) polymorphonuclear leukocytes (PMN's)
(b) lymphocytes, macrophages
(c) HLA-D; HLA-A, HLA-B, and HLA-C
(d) immunodeficiency; infections

Chapter 7

7–1 (a) False. In chronic granulomatous disease Fc receptors are intact; lysosomal enzyme functions are defective.
(b) True
(c) True
(d) False. SLE kidney disease is caused by complement-fixing immune complexes, not by the IgE system.
(e) False. Contact sensitivity is a manifestation of cellular immunity.
(f) True
(g) True
(h) False. ALS affects circulating T cells predominantly, although it may affect circulating B cells if the serum is not completely specific due to improper absorption. ALS treatment does not remove long-lived antibodies.
(i) False. These patients have a combined T-cell and B-cell immune system defect.
(j) False. It is linked to the human MHC, the HLA locus.

7–2 (a) T, B
(b) IgM; IgG immunoglobulins
(c) IgE; mast cells
(d) Goodpasture's syndrome
(e) mast (or B_ε)
(f) Hereditary angioneurotic edema
(g) T-cell (or cellular immunity)
(h) T
(i) bacterial
(j) immune complexes

Chapter 8

8–1 (a) False. Many normal cells divide more rapidly than most cancer cells (e.g., cells of the gastrointestinal tract and bone marrow). Tumor growth occurs because cancer cell division is not regulated and because generally both daughters of a cancer cell are capable of generating more cancer cells.

(b) False. If fetal components disappear before the maturation of the immune response (in most animals at or near birth), these components will in later life be recognized as foreign. In order to maintain a state of tolerance, components must generally be exposed to the immune system throughout the individual's life.

(c) False. Metastasis is the property of cancer *cells* to move from one site to another, resulting in tumor cell colonization of the second site.

(d) True

(e) True

(f) True. This observation suggests that at least some of the tumor-associated antigens are similar if not identical.

8-2 (a)   tumor-associated antigens
     (b)   suppress
     (c)   RNA-dependent DNA polymerase (reverse transcriptase)
     (d)   antigenic modulation
     (e)   surveillance
     (f)   plasma membrane
     (g)   Blocking factors

Index

159